# *Fear-Free*
# DENTAL CARE

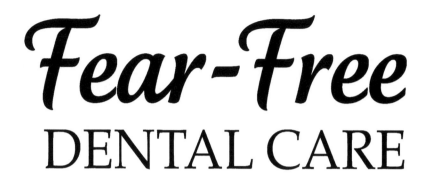

# Fear-Free
## DENTAL CARE

Finding a Dentist
You Can **LOVE**

DR. SCOTT SHAMBLOTT

Printed in the United States of America.

Dental Education Press, LLC
33 10th Avenue South, Suite 250
Hopkins, MN 55343
952-935-5599

Fear-Free Dental Care: Finding a Dentist You Can Love by Dr. Scott Shamblott

Editorial assistance: Bev Bachel
Design and layout: Aimee Libby

ISBN: 978-0-9791833-3-1

To my wife Kate and my daughter Rachel,
thanks for lighting up my life.

To my assistant Amy Knoll and
the entire Shamblott Family Dentistry staff,
thanks for brightening up my practice
and the lives of all our patients.

# Table of Contents

# Mission

At Shamblott Family Dentistry, we welcome all patients. Whether you see a dentist regularly or have avoided seeing one for many years, we will make you feel at home. We provide fear-free dental care while creating a pain-free, shame-free experience. We focus on your wants and needs to help take care of your health, using the most advanced techniques, technologies, and materials. Every patient leaves our office happy and smiling.

**Shamblott Family Dentistry**
33 10th Avenue South, Suite 250
Hopkins, MN 55343
952-935-5599
www.shamblottfamilydentistry.com

# Welcome

Are you afraid of going to the dentist?

If you're reading this book, you probably are. You're not alone. More than 80 percent of new patients who come to my office experience at least some degree of dental anxiety or fear. Some even suffer from a more serious condition: dental phobia.

Dental phobia is a legitimate condition suffered by millions of people in every society. In my practice, I see it every day. It affects both men and women of all ages and socio-economic groups. It has no respect for race, religion, or achievement, and the health consequences it causes require billions of dollars of treatment every year.

For those affected by this debilitating condition, it can feel like a bottomless pit of despair from which there is no escape. Yet, many who once suffered from dental phobia have found a way out.

Sound too good to be true? Well, then how did:

- Andrew go from avoiding the dentist for nearly two decades to flying halfway across the country for routine checkups?

- Steve, who wanted braces his entire adult life, work up the courage to finally take the first step by having his wisdom teeth pulled?

- Renata learn to control her panic so she wouldn't pass her dental fear on to her kids?

- Carol go from being afraid to walk into my office to laughing while in the waiting room?

- Susan turn a personal tragedy into an act of bravery that enabled her to realize her lifelong dream of having a perfect smile?

They did it the same way you can: by finding a dentist they could love.

That's exactly what this book will teach you how to do. It features everything I've learned during nearly two decades of practicing fear-free dental care. It also features the wisdom of many of my colleagues and other well-regarded experts in a variety of fields.

What it doesn't feature is constant reminders to brush twice daily, floss regularly, or schedule regular dental exams. Unless you've been living under a rock all your life, you already know these things are important.

Instead, you'll find success stories of real people whose anxiety, fear, and dental phobia kept them from seeing a dentist. Some of these men and women lived with mind-numbing pain for years. Others did so for decades. But now, thanks to my fear-free, pain-free approach to dental care, these same individuals see me regularly and get the dental care they need—and deserve. They beat their dental phobia, and believe me, if they could, so can you!

## What is Fear-Free Dental Care?

Put simply, fear-free dental care is a unique approach to dentistry that puts you and your needs front and center. Dentists who practice fear-free dental care focus on creating a kinder, gentler experience that makes it possible for even the most fearful patients to get the dental care they need. We do this by:

✔ Offering a variety of sedation options, including nitrous oxide laughing gas and IV sedation

✔ Using the most advanced tools, techniques, and materials

✔ Incorporating the latest scientific and psychological research

✔ Taking extra time to get to know you and your concerns

✔ Making sure you feel seen, heard, and respected

✔ Treating you with care and compassion

✔ Replacing judgment with empathy

- ✔ Putting the control where it belongs: in your hands

- ✔ Replacing shame-based lectures with proven anxiety-reducing techniques

- ✔ Fostering relationships based on trust, not authority

## I Can Help You

The principles of fear-free dental care work.

How do I know? Because I see the results every day: in the laughter I hear in my waiting room, in the relieved looks of patients as they leave my office, in the grateful smiles of those who are free of pain for the first time in a long, long time.

For nearly two decades, I've cared for thousands of patients, many of whom once went to great lengths to avoid seeing the dentist. I've witnessed the many ways dental fear, anxiety, and phobia manifest themselves. I've also learned firsthand how best to care for patients, no matter how anxious, fearful, or phobic they feel.

My fear-free, pain-free approach to dental care can help you, too. So thanks for picking up this book. By doing so you've taken an important first step toward beating dental phobia and taming your anxiety and fear. And now that you've taken that first step, are you ready to take another? Read on.

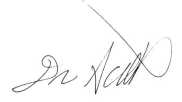

P.S. If you would like to schedule an appointment or simply talk with me or my staff about fear-free dental care, call my office at 952-935-5599. And if I'm not the right dentist for you for whatever reason, take the words of my daughter Rachel to heart: "If you don't see my dad, please see another dentist. Take care of your teeth because they're the only ones you get."

## DENTAL EMERGENCIES: ORDER YOUR FREE BOOK NOW

Ever had a tooth crack or a filling fall out? Ever had trouble falling asleep or been awakened in the middle of the night by a toothache? If so, you may benefit from my next book, which is about dental emergencies. To pre-order a FREE copy, call 952-935-5599 or send an email with your mailing address to book@shamblott.com.

# A Patient's Perspective

Perhaps you have experienced that there are people who come into our lives for the right reason at the right time. Dr. Scott Shamblott was not just the right dentist for me, he was the right man. We grew in our understanding of dental phobia together. I would probably be wearing dentures without him.

Not a day goes by when I don't think about dentistry. Every time I brush and floss—and every time I don't—I do it or DON'T do it contemplating how much I hate going to the dentist. Some people have a nonchalance about dentistry in the same way that they would about automotive maintenance. It's just something you have to do, right? Not to me. As a dental phobic, nothing is routine about dental care.

On one level, I understand how ridiculous that is. Can you imagine that before you take your car in for an oil change and a tune-up, you have to pray that your vehicle is going to come out of it all right or that superstitious rituals, such as washing your car in a certain way, will somehow help? Dental phobia is that irrational—and that real.

Great dentists like Dr. Scott Shamblott and dental phobic-friendly techniques can make a difference. Having a healthy, functional set of teeth is as important as good automotive maintenance; having a patient dentist allowed me to be a dental patient. If it's uncomfortable for you to eat or embarrassing when you smile, and you suspect that dental phobia is playing a part in a downward spiral of dental health, take some time to read this book and consider that there are alternatives, and that you are not alone.

Ian Punnett
*Patient, author, and radio broadcaster*

# THERE *IS* AN ALTERNATIVE

# Why People Fear The Dentist

*"The first step in solving a problem is to recognize that it does exist."*
— *Zig Ziglar, author and motivational speaker*

Very often I learn that a patient's fear of the dentist is something that runs in his or her family. Take Andrew, for instance. Like his mother, he's always had sensitive teeth, which meant suffering through pain-filled dental appointments—even as a child. After several particularly pain-filled ones while in junior and senior high school, he started avoiding his dentist altogether, something that became even easier for Andrew to do once he headed off to college. Avoiding the dentist was also easy for Andrew because he'd grown up seeing his mother do the exact same thing.

Before long, ten years had passed since Andrew had been to a dentist. He knew he should schedule an appointment, but just thinking about it made his heart race. Even seeing or hearing a dental drill on TV was enough to trigger his fear.

Things began to change for Andrew when his mother called him to say she had both good and bad news. The good news was that she'd finally conquered her fear and been to see a dentist. The bad news was that she needed a lot of dental work. A lot.

Worried that he was already in the same boat or soon would be, Andrew got serious about researching dentists. That's when he learned about IV sedation dentistry, a form of fear-free, pain-free dental care that I offer to patients who feel anxious or suffer from dental phobia.

While Andrew thought IV sedation dentistry could be a good option for him, he still put off making an appointment. Finally, the pain of a small crack in one of his back teeth became unbearable, and Andrew called my office. As my team and I try to do with all patients in pain, we asked Andrew to come in right away for a free consultation. He did, and three days later, I fixed his tooth. Not long after, Andrew was back. This time—thanks to the help of IV sedation—he had the rest of this teeth repaired and his wisdom teeth pulled.

Andrew's experience was so positive that even though he now lives in Santa Monica, California, he still comes to my Hopkins, Minnesota, office regularly for routine checkups and cleanings.

How did Andrew go from fearful to fearless? Partly, it was hearing the stories I told him about other patients who were in the same or worse situations. He realized that if they could get past their fear and conquer their dental phobia, he could, too. Andrew told me: "If IV sedation dentistry worked for them, it could work for me."

If you're like Andrew (and his mom), you fear—and perhaps even avoid—seeing the dentist. If so, you're not alone. Many people would rather do just about anything than walk into a dentist's office. I've even heard people say they would rather lose an arm or leg than have a root canal or a cavity filled. I don't take it personally. Instead, my heart goes out to these people. Clearly, they haven't found the right dentist.

But even people who have a dentist they love can still avoid seeing the dentist. In fact, I recently read a Consumers' Checkbook/Center for Study of Services article that stated that nervousness or anxiety about pain has led about 30 percent of people to avoid visiting a dentist for as long as possible at least once. WebMD reports that between 9 percent and 20 percent of Americans avoid going to the dentist because of anxiety or fear. The *Journal of the American Dental Association* estimates that ninety-two million Americans are afraid to get the dental work they need. And as I've already mentioned in my welcome, at least 80 percent of the new patients I see experience at least some degree of dental fear.

For my patients who suffer from full-blown dental phobia, that fear and anxiety builds up and can even lead to panic attacks. A panic attack is a sudden feeling of acute and disabling anxiety that can cause intense feelings of apprehension, fear, and impending doom. Such attacks can come on without warning. Symptoms include a racing heart, a rapid pulse, sweating, and feeling faint or light-headed.

> *A panic attack is a sudden feeling of acute and disabling anxiety that can cause intense feelings of apprehension, fear, and impending doom.*

If you've ever experienced a panic attack, you have plenty of company. Here's how comedian Amy Poehler describes her panic attacks in her book, *Yes Please:* "The best way I can explain a panic attack is that it's the feeling of someone inside my body stacking it with books. The books continue to pile up, and they make me feel like I can't breathe." Amy is one of many celebrities who acknowledge dealing with panic attacks. Others who do so include singer Donny Osmond, actress Kim Basinger, and media mogul Oprah Winfrey.

## Reasons Why People Avoid the Dentist

People avoid the dentist for many reasons. Some stem from very specific kinds of fear or phobias. Here are five of them:

### 1) Fear of Pain

"Is it going to hurt?" That's usually the first question patients ask me. Who can blame them? No one wants to feel even minor discomfort, let alone major pain. But given today's advanced technology, even serious dental issues can be addressed painlessly when handled the correct way.

## 2) Fear of Needles

Sometimes referred to as needle phobia, this is the fear of receiving an injection such as Novocain for numbing pain or antibiotics for fighting infection. Healthline estimates that a whopping 20 percent of people have a fear of needles.

## 3) Fear of Germs

Some people who avoid the dentist do so because they're afraid of germs. But proper sterilization of equipment kills all germs that can cause serious problems. Risk of germs is also reduced by the masks, gloves, and other protective clothing dentists and their staff are required to wear.

## 4) Fear of Drills

A lot of people hate the sound of my dental drill. I'm sure many even secretly wish I would turn it on myself, which reminds me of what former late-night talk-show host Johnny Carson once said: "Happiness is your dentist telling you it won't hurt a bit and then having him catch his hand in the drill." But seriously, the very sound of a dental drill is enough to cause many people anxiety.

### SHHHHHH

Today's drills are much quieter than previous ones. Some of my patients even report being able to block the sound of my drill entirely and relax completely when listening to music while wearing headphones. Perhaps Bob Marley was right when he said, "One good thing about music, when it hits you, you feel no pain."

## 5) Fear of the Unknown

Many people are made fearful of the dentist by a lack of knowledge of the treatment and processes involved. Take Art, for example. His dental anxiety stems from a fear of the unknown that began when he was a child. He once told me that he felt like the dentists he saw then did whatever they wanted, without ever explaining what they had planned or giving Art a choice.

As a result, once Art grew up, he made his own choice: he chose to stop going to the dentist. But that didn't stop his dental anxiety, which got worse with each passing year. Eventually Art's lack of dental care caught up with him, and he went in search of a fear-free dentist.

His search led him to me, and Art is glad it did. I took Art's fear of the unknown seriously and talked him through every step of what I planned to do ahead of time so he would know exactly what to expect. "You spent a lot of time talking with me upfront which helped ease my anxiety," says Art.

Here are other reasons why people avoid visiting the dentist:

**Sights, Sounds, and Tastes**
Even those who don't experience any of the previously listed fears sometimes report feeling hypersensitive to the sights, sounds, and smells of dental environments. Some dislike seeing the instruments. Others hate hearing the sound of plaque being scraped from their teeth. Still others are made queasy by the smell of antiseptic. While dentists can't turn their offices into sensory-free zones, most of us try to use warm lighting and calming music.

## SENSITIVE?

If the sights, sounds, and tastes of dentistry get the best of you, these tips can help:

- ✔ If you're sensitive to sights, keep your eyes closed or ask your dentist for a sleep mask or DVD glasses.

- ✔ If you're sensitive to sounds, wear headphones and listen to music or watch a movie.

- ✔ If you're sensitive to tastes, ask your dentist or hygienist to rinse your mouth frequently.

### Bad Memories

It's a fact: our brains are wired to help us avoid pain. As a result, bad memories stick around longer than good ones, which is why so many people can recall even minor dental pain long after the fact. Childhood memories can be particularly traumatic, but even hearing stories of other people's experiences can be disturbing. Take Bev, for instance. She was scared of having her wisdom teeth removed, not because she'd had a bad dental experience, but because she could recall so many horror stories of others who had.

## FORM NEW MEMORIES

The *primacy* effect means that we tend to better remember what we learn first rather than what we learn later. For example, let's say that your first dental experience was painful. The memory of that pain is likely to stick with you, even though subsequent appointments may be far more pleasant.

However, one thing trumps the primacy effect: the *recency* effect. This effect means we tend to better remember recent experiences than past ones, which is why a pleasant, pain-free dental appointment today will dull and even replace the memory of a less-than-pleasant childhood one, much the same way a newly saved document on the computer replaces a previous version.

### Cost

Yes, dental care costs money, and many people live within tight budgets. But for those suffering dental phobia, the cost of dental care can serve as an easy excuse. Some of the same people who hate spending their hard-earned money on dental care don't mind spending it on nice- but not need-to-haves such as lattes, manicures, or high-tech gadgets. While these things can be satisfying today, they pale in importance when compared to a person's ongoing health.

## A BITE OUT OF YOUR BUDGET

The truth of the matter is that taking care of your teeth and visiting your dentist regularly now can save you money in the long run: a small filling costs about $150 while putting off that filling could result in a root canal and crown that costs about $2,000. And the lifetime cost of a missing tooth? It could be as high as $25,000.

## No or Inadequate Insurance

Like access to health care, poor access to dental care is a national problem, one compounded by lack of insurance. According to one National Association of Dental Plans estimate I saw recently, more than 126 million Americans lack dental coverage (that's 2.67 times more than the number of Americans without medical coverage). According to another estimate, more than 44 percent of people don't go to the dentist because they have no coverage or insufficient coverage.

## DENTAL BENEFITS MATTER

According to the National Association of Dental Plans, people without dental benefits report higher incidences of illness and are:

✔ 67 percent more likely to have heart disease

✔ 50 percent more likely to have osteoporosis

✔ 29 percent more likely to have diabetes

## Dislike of Lectures

"If only you'd come in earlier." "You really need to floss." "Shame on you." Honestly, shame on all dentists, assistants, and hygienists who talk this way to their patients! Seriously.

If you already feel bad, guilty, or embarrassed by your dental health, the last thing you need is a dental professional who makes you feel bad about yourself, your teeth, or your dental habits. Regardless of how long it's been since you've seen a dentist or whether you brush and floss regularly or not at all, you don't deserve to be scolded, chastised, embarrassed, or humiliated in any way. Ever!

### Invasiveness

Like the classic video game that jumpstarted the modern gaming industry, some patients consider dentists to be "space invaders." That's because we not only get in your face, we get in your mouth. And mouths, despite being on public display, are one of our most private spaces.

> *You don't deserve to be scolded, chastised, embarrassed, or humiliated in any way. Ever!*

### Loss of Control

Some people feel an overwhelming sense of helplessness when in the dentist's chair because someone else is in control. This loss of control can be intensified by the feeling that personal space is being invaded.

### The Sterile, Impersonal Environment

The sterile and impersonal feel of some dental offices can distress patients, who may be further upset by the masks, gloves, and other protective clothing worn by dentists and their staff members. Combine this with the feeling of being treated like a number rather than an individual person with unique needs, and no wonder patients feel anxious.

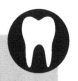

## WHAT'S BEHIND THE FEAR?

Here are five assumptions many people make about dental care that may be feeding into their fears. If these sound familiar to you, now's the perfect time to challenge these assumptions. Take the first step today by making an appointment with a dentist who practices fear-free dental care.

**FAULTY ASSUMPTION # 1:** All dentists are the same.

**FAULTY ASSUMPTION # 2:** I will always feel afraid.

**FAULTY ASSUMPTION # 3:** They're just teeth.

**FAULTY ASSUMPTION # 4:** All needed dental work must be completed at once.

**FAULTY ASSUMPTION # 5:** The pain will go away on its own.

# CHAPTER 2 | Fighting Fear with Knowledge

*"I will face my fear. I will permit it to pass over me and through me. And when it has gone past I will turn the inner eye to see its path. Where the fear has gone there will be nothing. Only I will remain."*
— *Frank Herbert, author of* Dune

**Mild Concern > Worry > Anxiety > Acute Stress > Dental Phobia**

Dental fear is not black and white, nor does it come in one size. In my practice, I see an entire spectrum, ranging from mild concern to full-blown dental phobia. What's the difference? Basically, it's a matter of degree.

Here's an overview of how you might experience the various stages of the spectrum:

**Mild Concern**
Your six-month exam is scheduled for next week. While you're not dwelling on the upcoming appointment, it crosses your mind once or twice a day. When it does, you mostly think about how you're going to make up the missed time at work, but every now and again you think about having your teeth cleaned and hope it won't take long or hurt.

**Worry**
You begin thinking about your upcoming appointment more often. But now, instead of thinking about it in a neutral way, you start to fret about

everything that could go wrong. What if your dentist or hygienist is mad at you for not flossing more often? What if you have a lot of cavities? What if that fleeting pain you experienced last week means you're going to need a root canal and crown?

**Anxiety**

Now you're on alert. Murphy's Law, which states that whatever can go wrong will go wrong, is the lens through which you view your day—and your upcoming appointment. Even though it's still a week away, you're starting to feel on edge. And when you think about your appointment, your heart may beat faster, your palms may sweat, and your muscles may tense.

## WARNING SIGNS OF ANXIETY

Here are some ways anxiety shows up in our bodies:

✔ Heavy breathing

✔ Facial grimacing

✔ Sighing

✔ Pacing

✔ Restlessness

✔ Increased heart rate

✔ Sweaty or moist palms

✔ Feeling hot or chilled

✔ Dizziness

✔ Excessive talking

✔ Inability to sleep

✔ Multiple trips to the bathroom

✔ Forgotten or missed appointments

✔ Frequent cancellation of appointments

✔ Last-minute cancellation of appointments

If you exhibit three or more of these warning signs, be sure to let your dentist know you need special attention.

## Acute Stress

When anxiety increases, it can turn into fear and trigger a "fight or flight" response, which is your body's way of telling you that something dangerous has been detected. That danger may be real or imagined. Unfortunately, your body can't tell the difference, so it reacts as if the danger is real. You start breathing faster, your heart beats faster, and your muscles flood with adrenaline. And while these physical reactions make sense when you're faced with physical danger from which you may have to quickly flee (a lion in the jungle, for instance), they aren't particularly helpful when it comes to having a positive dental experience.

## Dental Phobia

According to the American Psychiatric Association, a phobia is when a person has an irrational and excessive fear of something. In the case of dental phobia, that fear is of the dentist. If you suffer from dental phobia, you may go years—even decades—without even considering making an appointment. As a result, your dental health, or lack thereof, may interfere with your ability to eat, enjoy life, and even function. For instance, your pain may be so great that you cancel a vacation or find it difficult to sleep. In some cases, dental phobia may even lead to more dangerous, life-threatening situations, such as infections, diabetes, or a heart attack.

> *According to the American Psychiatric Association, a phobia is when a person has an irrational and excessive fear of something. In the case of dental phobia, that fear is of the dentist.*

## Don't Let This Happen to You

If you suffer from dental phobia, you may have the best intentions of visiting your dentist, but as the saying goes, "The road to hell is paved with good intentions." While I don't believe for a minute that you or anyone else is hell bound, I do believe that many of us, including myself, often put off the very care we need. As a result, what starts out as a tiny issue becomes a bigger, more costly problem. Here's how:

**JANUARY**

You go in for an appointment and your dentist notices a pinpoint of decay on one of your molars. Your dentist tells you about it and advises you to schedule an appointment right away.

**FEBRUARY**

You think about making an appointment but never get around to it.

**MARCH**

You finally call to schedule an appointment; the earliest you can get in is May.

**APRIL**

A few weeks before your appointment, your boss schedules a team meeting that conflicts with your appointment. You decide to ask your boss to reschedule the meeting.

**MAY**

A few days before your appointment, you realize you never asked your boss to reschedule the meeting. You also realize that your bank account balance is lower than you thought. You call your dentist and cancel your appointment.

## JUNE

Despite your best intentions, it's now been nearly six months since your dentist first noticed the decay and you still haven't been back. You finally call to reschedule your appointment, only to discover that the earliest your dentist can see you is August.

## AUGUST

You wake up on the day of your dental appointment with a sore throat. You call and cancel your appointment.

## SEPTEMBER

You receive a postcard in the mail from your dentist, reminding you of the need to reschedule your appointment. To help yourself remember to do so, you pin the postcard to your bulletin board.

## NOVEMBER

You call to reschedule your appointment.

## DECEMBER

Nearly one year after your initial appointment, you finally see your dentist. That's the good news. The bad news is that the pinpoint of decay your dentist pointed out in January has grown to encompass the entire inside of your tooth. What could have been a simple $150 filling is now a major cavity that may require a root canal and crown, which could cost $2,000 or more.

# Managing Fear Whenever it Appears

One way to get a handle on your dental fear is by becoming more aware of when and where it manifests itself. Some people are most anxious in the weeks leading up to their appointment, others when they first arrive at their dentist's office, and still others after their appointment is over.

## Pre-Appointment Anxiety

If the very thought of an upcoming dental appointment stresses you out, you may suffer from pre-appointment anxiety. Many people are able to manage this anxiety, but some find it overwhelming, sometimes so much so that they repeatedly cancel their appointments.

If you suffer from pre-appointment anxiety, talk with your dentist and his or her staff several weeks before your appointment. Share your fears and concerns with them, and ask them for their help. Also consider enlisting the help of a trusted friend whom you can call whenever you start to feel nervous or on edge. You may also want to line up a "dental buddy" to go with you to your appointment. Sometimes just knowing that someone will be with you can help you feel less fearful and more relaxed.

The relaxation techniques in Chapter 11 and the apps on page 78 can also help.

## ATTACK YOUR PANIC

So many of my patients have confided that they've had panic attacks at some point in their lives, whether in anticipation of an appointment, during an appointment, or afterwards. If you suffer from such attacks, you are not alone! According to WebMD, more than 2.4 million U.S. adults experience panic attacks, and although the cause is often a mystery, here are some tips that can help:

**LEARN ABOUT PANIC.** Simply knowing more about panic, its symptoms, and how common it is, can go a long way toward relieving your anxiety. Visit www.webmd.com or www.mayoclinic.org to learn more.

**AVOID CIGARETTES AND CAFFEINE.** Smoking and caffeine can contribute to panic attacks in some people. If you're susceptible, avoid smoking and drinking coffee or other caffeinated beverages before seeing your dentist. Also be careful with non-drowsy cold medications and other medications that contain stimulants.

**CONTROL YOUR BREATHING.** Hyperventilating—a condition in which you suddenly start to breathe very quickly, exhaling more than you inhale—can bring on many of the symptoms associated with a panic attack. Slow, deep breathing can relieve the symptoms and help you calm down.

**PRACTICE RELAXATION.** When practiced regularly, the muscle relaxation technique on pages 77-78 can go a long way toward helping you counteract your panic. Activities such as yoga and meditation can help as well. These activities also come with a bonus: those who practice them regularly report feelings of joy and serenity.

## Post-Appointment Anxiety

Like all dentists, I hope that my patients experience a sense of relief after their visit. Unfortunately, some people continue to experience anxiety. This post-appointment anxiety can be just as debilitating as pre-appointment anxiety. It may also take many of the same forms—increased heart rate, sweaty palms, and inability to sleep, for example.

As opposed to those with pre-appointment anxiety who worry about what's going to happen, those who suffer from post-treatment anxiety worry about what has happened. Did they get the treatment they expected? The results they wanted? Did they experience more pain during treatment than they were prepared for? Were they surprised by seeing some blood? Were they treated with care and concern? What happened once the numbness wore off? The answers to any of these questions can cause additional fear and anxiety, bringing a patient full-circle back to the same level of anxiety experienced before the appointment.

Knowing what to expect after your appointment can lessen your fears and reduce your anxiety, which is why I always explain ahead of time exactly what patients should be prepared for once they leave my office. It's also why I always give written after-treatment instructions.

You can lessen your post-treatment anxiety—and more importantly, your post-treatment pain—by carefully following your dentist's instructions. If he tells you to rinse your mouth with salt water, do it. If she warns against eating solid foods or drinking alcohol, don't. If he tells you to relax and take it easy for the rest of the day, by all means, relax; doing so keeps your pulse rate low, which helps to promote healing and minimize both bleeding and swelling. And finally, if she says to ice a certain area for twenty minutes, then let it warm up for twenty minutes, and to repeat this cycle for three to four days, by all means, DO IT!

Your dentist should also give you a phone number to call if you have questions or concerns once you leave the office. I give my personal cell phone number to my patients so that they can call me directly if they have questions following a procedure. And, of course, my main office number is answered, even after hours.

> *Remember, pain is an important warning signal. If your pain becomes unbearable or stretches beyond what your dentist told you to expect, call your dentist immediately.*

Remember, pain is an important warning signal. If your pain becomes unbearable or stretches beyond what your dentist told you to expect, call your dentist immediately.

## PAIN PILLS: TAKE THE FIRST ONE WHILE YOU'RE STILL NUMB

If your dentist prescribes pain pills, taking the first one before your numbness wears off is one of the best ways to keep yourself pain-free.

# CHAPTER 3

# Dental Anxiety Self-Test

*"Keep smiling. It makes people wonder what you've been up to."*
— *Becky Fowler Blackmon, author*

Do you suffer from dental anxiety? Take this self-test developed by Dr. Norman Corah to find out.

Circle the most appropriate answer to each of the following multiple-choice questions. Then turn to page 23 to see how to score your answers.

## QUESTION 1

If you had to go to the dentist tomorrow, how would you feel about it?

a. I would look forward to it as a reasonably enjoyable experience.
b. I wouldn't care one way or the other.
c. I would be a little uneasy about it.
d. I would be afraid that it would be unpleasant and painful.
e. I would be very frightened of what the dentist might do.

## QUESTION 2

When you are waiting in the dental office for your turn in the chair, how do you feel?

a. Relaxed.
b. A little uneasy.

c. Tense.

d. Anxious.

e. So anxious that I sometimes break out in a sweat or almost feel physically sick.

# QUESTION 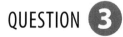 3

When you are in the dentist's chair waiting while he gets his drill ready to begin working on your teeth, how do you feel?

a. Relaxed.

b. A little uneasy.

c. Tense.

d. Anxious.

e. So anxious that I sometimes break out in a sweat or almost feel physically sick.

# QUESTION 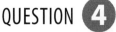 4

You are in the dentist's chair to have your teeth cleaned. While you are waiting and the dentist is getting out the instruments which he will use to scrape your teeth around the gums, how do you feel?

a. Relaxed.

b. A little uneasy.

c. Tense.

d. Anxious.

e. So anxious that I sometimes break out in a sweat or almost feel physically sick.

Corah NL: Development of a Dental Anxiety Scale. *Journal of Dental Research* 48:596, 1969.

## Scoring the Quiz

Give yourself:

**1** point for each a.

**2** points for each b.

**3** points for each c.

**4** points for each d.

**5** points for each e.

Now determine your anxiety level (there is a maximum of 20 points):

**FEWER THAN 9 POINTS** = little to no anxiety

**9-12 POINTS** = moderate anxiety

**13-14 POINTS** = high anxiety

**15-20 POINTS** = severe anxiety or dental phobia

# CHAPTER 4 | Finding A Dentist You Can Love

*"It's not about finding a dentist. It's about finding the right dentist."*

— *Karen Carlson, dental assistant*

Finding a dentist is an important decision for you and your family. After all, you'll be trusting an important part of your health to this person. And although many people simply poll their friends and family for a recommendation, you may want to take a more thoughtful approach, especially if you're among the ninety-two million Americans who feel anxious or fearful about seeing the dentist.

Here's the process I recommend:

## STEP 1

### Establish Criteria

Before you can find the right dentist, you have to know what's "right" for you. Here are some basic criteria to consider:

✔ **Location.** Do you want a dentist who's just around the corner from where you live or work or are you willing to drive across town to see the right dentist? For most people, keeping an appointment is easier when their dentist is nearby, but people with dental anxiety are willing to travel greater distances to see a fear-free, pain-free dentist. Some of my patients even fly halfway across the country to keep their appointments. Also think about how you will get to and from your appointments. Do you need a dentist who is on the bus line or one who offers free parking?

✔ **Hours.** Some dentists work Monday through Thursday 9 a.m. to 5 p.m. Others are open Fridays and Saturdays, as well as early mornings and evenings.

✔ **Specializations.** Dentists specialize in different things. For instance, I practice general dentistry with an emphasis on fear-free, pain-free dental care and sedation dentistry. Other dentists focus on cosmetic dentistry or specialize in orthodontics or oral surgery.

✔ **Features.** Do you need a dentist who offers nitrous oxide laughing gas or one who offers IV sedation? One who lets you watch videos or listen to music? One who speaks Spanish or is good with kids? One who has a wheelchair-accessible office or one with free parking? Knowing ahead of time which features matter to you will help you find a dentist who meets your needs—today and for the long run.

✔ **In-network provider.** Depending on whether or not you have dental insurance and the type of insurance you have, you may prefer a dentist who is a member of your network's plan.

✔ **Financing options.** Some dentists offer discount programs for patients who don't have insurance. For example, we offer Smile Savers, which gives patients a 15 percent discount on services performed at Shamblott Family Dentistry. We also give patients a range of financing options via programs such as CareCredit and Lending Club. For details on these and other programs, call my office at 952-935-5599.

## CHANGING DENTISTS

While having a long-term relationship with your dentist is just as important as having one with your doctor, there may come a time when you need to find a new dentist who is better suited to your needs. If so, don't feel guilty. People change dentists all the time.

If you decide to start seeing a new dentist, be sure to ask your old dentist for your patient chart, which you are legally entitled to. It contains a complete record of all your dental visits, including chart notes and any problems that have been identified. Also request your x-rays (although if it's been awhile since they were taken, expect your new dentist to order new x-rays during your first appointment).

## STEP

### Start Building a List

If you have dental insurance, your plan will provide a list of dentists who are part of the plan. Many insurers also offer a "Find a Dentist" tool on their websites, which you can use to search for a dentist by name, address, or specialty, as well as by the specific features such as "fear-free dental care" that you identified in Step 1.

Ask friends, family members, and coworkers for recommendations. Also use your social networks. A friend of a friend may say, "My dentist is great," giving you a recommendation you wouldn't have gotten any other way. Your family doctor or neighborhood pharmacist may have suggestions as well.

Many dentists advertise in local newspapers or on radio and TV. Some, like me, have even hosted radio programs. But remember to do your own research because not every dentist who advertises is adept at treating people with dental anxiety and fear.

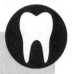

High-fear patients should be wary of retail chain clinics. While such clinics may seem a good option, they can be anything but. Patients are often assigned to a different hygienist or dentist each time, which makes it hard to develop trust. And because chain clinics typically focus on getting patients in and out quickly, they can be a nightmare for those who already fear seeing the dentist.

## STEP

### Learn More

Your dental plan's website is a great place to start your research, but don't stop there. Instead, call each dentist who seems like a good fit to gather additional information. Here are some questions to ask when you call (if you can't find the answers on the dentist's website):

✔ How long has the dentist been practicing?

✔ What specific credentials has the dentist earned?

✔ How does the dentist and the dental staff keep abreast of new developments?

✔ How far in advance do I need to book appointments?

✔ If I have an emergency, how quickly will I be able to see the dentist?

✔ How are emergencies handled outside of regular office hours?

✔ Does the dentist want to treat patients who are fearful, and does he or she have experience doing so?

✔ What steps does the dentist take in treating patients who are fearful?

✔ What are the office hours? Can I go before or after work or on the weekend?

✔ Does the dentist offer nitrous oxide laughing gas? Is there a charge for it?

✔ What type of anesthesia will the dentist administer to help me relax?

✔ What other tools does the dentist have available to help me relax?

✔ Will the dentist and the staff review my treatment options and costs with me ahead of time?

✔ What type of financing options does the dental office offer?

✔ Is there a discount program if I do not have dental insurance?

By asking questions such as these, you not only gather important information about the dentists you're considering and their practices, you also get clues as to how you'll be treated. A front-office staff that's knowledgeable, courteous, and willing to spend time on the phone answering your questions can go a long way toward putting you at ease.

Also, a staff that's willing to listen and respond to your needs *before* you're a patient is likely to treat you the same way *after* you're a patient. On the other hand, if a dentist's front-office staff leaves you on hold indefinitely or appears too rushed to answer your questions or address your concerns, it may be a sign that the dentist will do the same.

> *By asking questions such as these, you not only gather important information about the dentists you're considering and their practices, you also get clues as to how you'll be treated.*

# STEP

### Visit the Office

Once you've found a dentist that you believe may be right for you, visit his or her office. Is it easy enough to get to? Is the waiting room inviting? Are the people friendly? Do you feel comfortable there? Does anything you see, smell, or hear upset you? Can you imagine yourself as a patient?

Also use your visit to ask any additional questions you may have. You may even want to see if you can meet the dentist. While such spur-of-the-moment meetings aren't always possible, I and many other dentists who treat fearful patients understand how stressful choosing a dentist can be and will do all we can to put you at ease—even before you make your first appointment.

# STEP 5

### Schedule an Appointment

When scheduling your appointment, think about what time of day will work best for you. For instance, if you're a night owl, you may prefer an afternoon or evening appointment. On the other hand, if you're an early riser who would rather get your appointment out of the way, you may want to request the first appointment of the day. Also take into account the time of day you're most likely to feel relaxed.

# STEP 6

### Keep Your Appointment

If you fear the dentist, keeping your appointment can be a challenge. Make getting to your dentist's office the first hurdle you overcome. Many of my patients do this by enlisting someone to drive them to their appointments. Also, if you have a history of canceling appointments or procrastinating when it comes to making them, talk with your dentist or his or her staff. Once they understand that fear is driving your behavior, they will not only be more understanding, they will be able to offer more help.

# Stepping into Fear-Free Dental Care

*"My motto is: feel the fear and do it anyway."*
— *Tamara Mellon, cofounder of Jimmy Choo*

My patient Kathy's dental fears began after a series of anxiety-filled appointments with a dentist who caused her a lot of pain but never entirely fixed her problems. She eventually got so frustrated that she threw in the towel and called it quits. A few years later, in pain and more anxious than ever, Kathy came to see me. I'm so glad she did.

When I asked Kathy to think back on that first appointment with me and what felt so different from her previous dental experiences, I was delighted by what she had to say: "Everyone in your office is really caring and compassionate. I was scared to death. They understood that and took my concerns seriously. Thanks to them, I not only got through that first appointment, I've gotten through many more since."

If you suffer from dental fear or anxiety, finding the right office is important. And you should feel as if you have found it as soon as you step into the office. Here's a list of things to look for:

**A Pleasant Waiting Room**
When you walk into the dentist's office, you should feel as if you're entering a friendly, comfortable space.

**A Warm Greeting**
If you've had a bad dental experience or are afraid of seeing your dentist, what happens in the first few minutes of your appointment can go a long

way toward helping you relax. Even the way the receptionist says hello can play a role. Here are some examples of greetings that I think work well and that you can expect to hear from any dentist who takes a fear-free, pain-free approach to dental care:

- "Hi. It's great to see you again. Thanks for arriving on time. We really appreciate that and will do our best to get you on your way as quickly as possible."

- "Thanks for coming. We're right on schedule. Take a seat, but don't get too comfortable. We'll be calling your name in less than five minutes."

- "Welcome. I know it's your first time here, and I want to reassure you that you're in good hands. Your dentist is not only good at what she does, she's a great person. You're going to love her."

## Eye Contact

The eyes, often referred to as the "messengers of the soul," are important for establishing rapport. When your dentist, dental hygienist, and other members of your dental team make and maintain eye contact, they're showing you that they care and are interested in what you have to say and how you feel. On the other hand, if they ask you about your concerns and then look out the window or roll their eyes while you respond, they're telling you that their mind is elsewhere or that they think very little of you.

Eye contact is also important for another reason. By looking directly at you—and really seeing you, fears and all—your dentist gains important information about you. For instance, if you smile at his banter, he may sense that you're at ease, whereas if you grimace every time she mentions the word "plaque," she may realize that you're feeling anxious.

## An Interest in You

Your dentist should demonstrate an interest in who you are by asking you questions about what you like to do, whether that's reading books, watching movies, playing cards, knitting, skiing, traveling, or hanging out with your kids or grandkids. Such questions help develop a positive dentist-patient relationship. By getting to know you, your dentist can help keep the conversation flowing which, in turn, can ease your anxiety and help you relax. Dentists who are particularly adept conversationalists can even use conversation to help distract you.

## THE NAME GAME

Most dentists and their staff members will call you by your first name. However, if you prefer being addressed some other way, say so. Also, if what to call your dentist or how to pronounce his or her name is causing you anxiety, just ask. Some dentists prefer being addressed as Doctor So and So, while others prefer you use their first name as this can help establish a more equal, less threatening relationship right from the start.

**Clear Explanations**

All dentists and their staff members should provide clear explanations of exactly what you can expect to happen throughout your appointment. Doing so helps reduce your fear of the unknown. So do clear explanations of the sensations you can expect to experience.

Here are some examples of the types of comments you might hear from me or an assistant or hygienist in my office:

- "We'd like to take x-rays today. Are you okay with that?"

- "You might feel a slight pinch. It won't really hurt, but I don't want you to be surprised."

- "I'm just going to finish cleaning up this last little bit of decay. To do so, I'm swapping from a high-speed to low-speed drill. It won't be as noisy, but you may notice that it vibrates a bit more. The vibration won't cause any pain, but it will feel a bit different."

- "I'm going to rinse your mouth now. You'll feel the cool water soothing your gums. When I have work done on my teeth, this is always one of my favorite parts."

- "I'm getting ready to polish your teeth, which is why you can probably smell spearmint. That's the last step. After that, you're all done."

## DON'T BE AFRAID TO ASK

If your dentist or dental staff uses terms you don't understand, stop and ask that the information be repeated in easy-to-understand language that makes sense to you.

### Reassurance

When you're the patient, a little reassurance can go a long way toward helping you feel safe and secure, which is why it's so important for your dentist and hygienist to offer words of encouragement throughout your appointment. Not only do such words help relax you, they help distract you.

Here are some examples of the types of reassuring phrases you can expect to hear from dentists who take a fear-free, pain-free approach to dental care:

- "You're doing great."

- "I know this isn't easy for you, but it's going really well."

- "You should be proud of yourself for how well you're doing."

- "You can relax. Everything is going just as planned."

- "I was just thinking about how far you've come since your first visit. No wonder I'm smiling."

- "Congratulations. You've made it through the hardest part. It gets easier from here."

Throughout your appointment, your dentist should speak to you in a warm, friendly, confident tone. And while he or she should never speak too fast, which can make you feel as if you're being hurried along, most people appreciate dentists who demonstrate their passion. Dentists may do this by talking about similar procedures they've performed on others and the results achieved (although, in accordance with the Health Insurance Portability and Accountability Act, commonly referred to as HIPAA, your dentist should never reveal a patient's full name or other identifying circumstances).

Dentists may also demonstrate their concern for you by talking with you about things you enjoy or care deeply about: your family, pets, hobbies, the charities you support, where you're going on vacation, or, in my case, the eighties rock music I love. This "small talk" is important: it helps regulate anxiety.

## A Warranty
Most dentists are proud of the dentistry they provide. Many even offer warranties. For instance, my practice offers:

- ✔ A two-year warranty on dental sealants and composite (tooth-colored) fillings

- ✔ A three-year warranty on dentures and partial dentures

- ✔ A five-year warranty on crowns, bridges, inlays, onlays, and porcelain veneers

For a copy of our warranty, visit www.shamblottfamilydentistry.com and download the New Patient Form, which you'll find in the left column at the bottom of the home page. (Note: For our warranty to be active, you must return to our office to get your teeth cleaned and examined at least two times per year.)

# CHAPTER 6

# Qualities of Fear-Free Dentists

*"It's far more impressive when others discover your good qualities without your help."*
— *Judith Martin, Miss Manners and etiquette authority*

Moira is an adventurer. From scuba diving to hiking and camping, her passion for exploring has led her to many new experiences. But, after having several root canals, she knew dental pain was one experience she never wanted to explore again, which is why she came to see me. She started our appointment by explaining that it always takes her a long time to get numb or sedated. "I could be told to count to ten," Moira said, "and find myself at fifteen, wondering when I'm going to stop feeling or be knocked out."

Moira explained this to other dentists, yet many downplayed her concerns, often starting to treat her before ensuring she was completely numb. "They'd start full tilt and then hit an un-numbed nerve," says Moira. "It was excruciating."

Over time, Moira developed dental anxiety. For a while she even avoided dentists altogether, but her pain eventually drove her back. She then had two root canals in six months, both painful, and knew something had to change. She told me she just couldn't take it anymore. That's when her partner recommended she see me. Reluctantly, Moira agreed to do so.

With just one look in Moira's mouth, I was able to tell her why she had needed so many root canals—because she grinds her teeth, which over time causes teeth to crack. No other dentist, including the specialists Moira had seen, had ever mentioned that as the cause of her many root canals.

I was also able to pinpoint the primary reason it takes Moira so long to get numb. It's because she has two nerves that go to her back teeth; most people have only one. Some dentists don't have the patience to wait for patients like Moira to get numb, but I do, which Moira acknowledged when she shared the following: "I never feel that you're watching the clock or trying to rush me in and out. And you never assume I'm numb. Instead, you test again and again to make sure I am."

*I never feel that you're watching the clock or trying to rush me in and out. And you never assume I'm numb. Instead, you test again and again to make sure I am.*

It makes me so happy when patients like Moira thank me for being careful and attentive because skills needed to care for "the whole patient" are something I've worked to develop in my practice. They're also a cornerstone of my fear-free, pain-free approach to dental care.

Here are some other qualities that can help you identify whether your dentist practices fear-free, pain-free dental care:

## Fear-Free Dentists Listen

Your dentist should be good at asking questions. He or she should also be good at listening to your answers because the best questions aren't yes or no questions, but open-ended questions such as:

- What brought you here today?

- How can I help you?

- How can I make this appointment or procedure easier for you?

All of these questions and others like them give you the chance to talk about what's on the top of your mind and encourage you to share whatever you feel most like talking about.

Here's an example of how a conversation with a fear-free dentist might go:

| THE DENTIST: | SAYS: |
| --- | --- |
| *Acknowledges your anxiety* | "I understand you're feeling apprehensive about today's appointment, perhaps even a little afraid. What can you tell me about how you're feeling?" |
| *Engages you in conversation* | "I'm sorry you've had bad experiences in the past. I can only imagine how difficult this must be. What can I do to make this appointment easier for you?" |
| *Explores your concerns* | "Great. I really want to understand your concerns. What can you tell me about your past dental experiences and how they contribute to your fear and anxiety?" |
| *Restates the problem* | "Thanks for sharing with me. I'd like to recap what you just said to make sure I have a clear understanding of your current situation as well as your concerns. Is it okay if I go ahead?" |
| *Offers a solution* | "Now that I have a clear understanding of the problem and your concerns, I'd like to share what I recommend in terms of how we can best proceed without triggering your fear and anxiety. Are you ready for that?" |

Notice how each step of the consultation ends with a question. Questions give you the opportunity to tell your story in your own way, which helps you feel more in control.

## Fear-Free Dentists Move from Generalities to Specifics

Throughout this exchange of information—which should feel like an everyday conversation—the dentist will be listening to what you say (for example, "I haven't been to the dentist in fifteen years") and to what you don't say (for example, "I'm afraid"). The dentist will also be paying attention to other aspects of your verbal communication (for example, your tone and how fast you talk), as well as your nonverbal communication (for example, your facial expressions and whether you're sitting still or fidgeting).

Your dentist, who should be doing more listening than talking, will be working to keep a two-way conversation going. He or she will also be encouraging you to move from general statements to more specific ones in order to identify the origin of your fear. Here are two examples of why moving to specifics is so important to the care your fear-free, pain-free dentist provides:

# EXAMPLE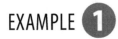

**General statement:**
I don't like the dentist.

**Specific statement:**
Well really, it's the drill I hate.

**Origin-of-fear statement:**
When I was seven or eight years old, the dentist dropped the drill on my lip and it really hurt. And when I started to cry, he laughed and told me I was too old to be acting like such a big baby. I felt so humiliated. I didn't even tell my mom what happened. And ever since, just hearing the drill makes my heart race.

**How a fear-free dentist can help:**
Now that the dentist knows that it's the sound of the drill that bothers you, he or she can offer you earplugs so you can block out the sound or headphones so you can listen to music.

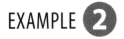

**General statement:**

I'm worried I'll faint.

**Specific statement:**

I sometimes faint when I get nervous.

**Origin-of-fear statement:**

The last time I got my teeth cleaned, I fainted. One minute I was taking off my jacket and the next I was waking up on the floor. Everyone was so concerned. They wanted to know if they should call an ambulance. I felt really stupid. Now, I am more nervous than ever.

**How a fear-free dentist can help:**

Now that the dentist knows why you feel anxious, he or she can help you relax by talking to you, distracting you, and perhaps even offering you nitrous oxide laughing gas.

## Fear-Free Dentists Use Positive Language

A fear-free dentist always uses language that comes across as positive and constructive, rather than language that causes fear and anxiety. This reminds me of one of my favorite cartoons. The scene is a dental school. There's an anxious-looking patient in the dental chair, and a student dentist and teacher standing by his side. The teacher advises the student, "Instead of 'You're entering a world of pain,' try 'This won't hurt a bit.'"

> **" A fear-free dentist always uses language that comes across as positive and constructive, rather than language that causes fear and anxiety. "**

Here are some other examples of how I and other fear-free dentists reframe negative language into language that is more positive and affirming:

| NEGATIVE LANGUAGE: | POSITIVE LANGUAGE: |
|---|---|
| This won't hurt. | I don't expect you to feel anything. |
| This may hurt. | You will feel a bit of pressure. |
| I'll be giving you a shot now. | I'll be numbing your gum now. You'll feel a slight poke. |
| I'm going to pull your tooth now. | I'm going to remove your tooth now. |
| You may feel some pain. | You shouldn't feel any pain. But if you do, or if you feel the least bit uncomfortable, raise your hand and I'll stop immediately. |

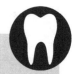

## BODY LANGUAGE SPEAKS VOLUMES

If the tone of your dentist's voice and body language—posture, movement, gestures, eye contact, and facial expressions—doesn't match his or her words, you may want to consider finding a different dentist. That's because body languages makes up 55 percent of what a person communicates, while tone makes up 38 percent and words only 7 percent.

Also be aware that your body language gives your dentist important clues as to the presence and level of anxiety you're experiencing. For instance, if you start breathing rapidly or sweating profusely, your body is telling your dentist that you feel anxious, perhaps even afraid. And if you keep your feet hanging off the chair or move around a lot, you may be communicating that you are psychologically preparing to flee.

## Fear-Free Dentists Are Honest—But Never Shaming

Your dentist and all members of his or her team should be honest at all times. By doing so, they earn your trust. And the more you trust them, the less anxious you'll feel.

While trust takes time to earn, it can be lost in a nanosecond, which is why most dentists work so hard to tell you the truth, even if it's not what you want to hear. But keep in mind that even news you don't want to hear can be delivered in a good way.

For instance, it's okay for dentists to say, "You have five cavities."

It's not okay for them to say, "I told you that if you didn't start flossing you'd end up with cavities."

> *While trust takes time to earn, it can be lost in a nanosecond, which is why most dentists work so hard to tell you the truth, even if it's not what you want to hear. But keep in mind that even news you don't want to hear can be delivered in a good way.*

Dentists also need to speak honestly about the treatment you need and the fees associated with that treatment. Saying you need one filling and then doing three is unacceptable, as is telling you the cost is $250 and then charging you $500. That said, while treating you, your dentist may discover that you need more work than he or she originally thought. Even so, he or she still needs your approval for the extra work. You should never be surprised by a bigger-than-expected bill.

Also expect your dentist to respond honestly to your nonverbal signals. For instance, if you flinch, even slightly, your dentist shouldn't pretend not to have noticed. Instead, your dentist should acknowledge what happened and respond accordingly: "Are you okay? I saw you tense a little. That must mean you felt a little something. Did you? Because if you did, I can do something to fix that." As I tell all my patients, "No suffering, unless it's something you really want to do."

You also need to be honest with your dentist. Tell him or her about all medical conditions, as well as all operations and surgical procedures. Also disclose all the medications you take, including any over-the-counter medications, supplements, and herbal supplements, as well as any recreational or illegal drug use. Such disclosure is in your best interest. Without it, your dentist could recommend a treatment or prescribe a medication that harms rather than helps.

> *You also need to be honest with your dentist. Tell him or her about all medical conditions, as well as all operations and surgical procedures.*

## Fear-Free Dentists Offer Options

Just as one size doesn't fit all when it comes to dental fear, neither does one size fit all when it comes to helping people deal with their fear. In fact, a solution that works for one person may have just the opposite effect on another. And a solution that works for one person today may not work for that same person tomorrow.

That's why a true fear-free, pain-free dentist offers a variety of options. Which option is right for you depends on where you fall on the fear spectrum: the greater, more debilitating your fear and anxiety, the more robust the solution you'll want to consider.

For an overview of the pain-free options offered by fear-free, pain-free dentists, see Chapter 8.

## Fear-Free Dentists Empower Their Patients

For many people who fear the dentist or experience dental anxiety, a main concern is lack of control. They want to be able to answer the question, "What if?"

- What if I need to swallow?

- What if I have to go to the restroom?

- What if I want to ask a question?

- What if I need you to STOP what you're doing…RIGHT NOW?

One way you can have control is by asking your dentist to agree on a signal that means "stop" that you can use whenever you feel you need a break or are feeling even the smallest amount of discomfort. I often tell my patients,

"I don't expect you to feel any pain, but if you do or if you want to stop for any reason, just raise your hand and I'll stop as fast as I can."

The important thing isn't the signal itself but what happens when you give the signal. A fear-free, pain-free dentist will stop immediately. Not when he feels like it, not when she finishes what she's doing, not in three seconds, but now. Right now!

## FIND YOUR MATCH

If you don't feel comfortable with the dental hygienist assigned to you, ask for another one. That's one of the ways my patient Carol took control of her dental care. "When I first went to see Dr. Shamblott, the hygienist assigned to me was both strong and strong-willed," says Carol. "That intimidated me, so I asked for someone else." The hygienist Carol sees now is outwardly warmer and more nurturing, which works better for Carol.

## Fear-Free Dentists Have a Gentle Touch

Touch matters, often more than you think. One reason is because the sense of touch is located in your skin, which covers your entire body. Contrast this with your other four senses (sight, hearing, smell, and taste), which are located in specific parts of your body (eyes, ears, nose, and mouth).

Obviously you should expect your dentist to treat your mouth and your teeth with care, only exerting as much pressure as is needed. You may also notice that your dentist and others in his or her office reach out to touch you in other ways. That's because a hand squeeze or a shoulder touch can go a long way in helping you feel relaxed and cared for.

## FINDING A DENTIST YOU CAN LOVE

Here's how some people explain how they knew they'd found the dentist who was right for them:

> "You fly from Santa Monica to Minneapolis just to have your teeth cleaned."
> - *Andrew*

> "You recommend your dentist to people you care about, even your boss."
> - *Kris*

> "You'd rather see your dentist than live with the pain."
> - *Steve*

> "You no longer shake like a leaf when you pull into the parking lot."
> - *Adam*

> "You can have your teeth cleaned without nitrous oxide laughing gas."
> - *Laura*

> "You don't have to pay for your initial appointment or first set of x-rays."
> - *Moira*

> "You get a couple of prescriptions the night before so that you sleep better and are less anxious. Then you come in and get sedated by a Certified Registered Nurse Anesthetist. You feel nothing, you remember nothing. It's great."
> - *Lisa*

CHAPTER

# 7 | Your Rights and Responsibilities

*"The earth is the mother of all people, and all people should have equal rights upon it."*

— *Chief Joseph, leader of the Wallowa Native American tribe*

Once upon a time, doctors and dentists knew best. They acted from on high, and their recommendations were never questioned. Times have changed. Today, people want and deserve relationships that are built on mutual trust and respect.

Like all successful relationships, your relationship with your dentist requires both parties working together. While you need to decide for yourself what you want in a relationship with your dentist, here are some of the qualities most of my patients consider important:

✔ Respect

✔ Compassion

✔ Communication

✔ Honesty

✔ Trust

✔ Follow-through

## Patient Bill of Rights

As a patient, you have rights. These rights guarantee you accurate information, fair treatment, and the ability to make your own decisions. While each dentist's bill of rights is unique, most are similar to the Shamblott Family Dentistry Patient Bill of Rights, which you'll find below.

Most dentists post their bill of rights on their website and in their waiting rooms. You can also request a copy.

### SHAMBLOTT FAMILY DENTISTRY PATIENT BILL OF RIGHTS

As a patient of Shamblott Family Dentistry, you have the right to:

✔ See the dentist and hygienist of your choice.

✔ See the same dentist and hygienist every time you receive dental treatment.

✔ Be told in advance the type of treatment you need and what it will cost.

✔ Ask about treatment alternatives and be told the advantages and disadvantages of each in language you can understand.

✔ Expect your dentist and all members of his or her team to keep you safe.

✔ Know the education and training of your dentist and his or her team.

# Patient Responsibilities

In addition to having rights, you also have responsibilities. Some common patient responsibilities are summarized below.

As a patient you will, to the best of your ability:

- ✔ Provide honest, accurate, and complete information about your present and past health, including current complaints, recent illnesses, and all medications you take.

- ✔ Inform your dentist if you don't understand the recommended course of treatment.

- ✔ Follow your dentist's instructions.

- ✔ Accept responsibility for your actions if you refuse treatment or opt not to follow your dentist's instructions.

- ✔ Keep appointments and, when unable to do so, notify your dentist in a timely manner.

- ✔ Pay for your treatment in a timely manner per office policy.

PART

# EXPERIENCING FEAR-FREE DENTAL CARE

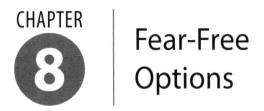

# CHAPTER 8 | Fear-Free Options

*"Find a place inside where there's joy, and the joy will burn out the pain."*

*— Joseph Campbell, mythologist and writer*

Ian, who wrote the patient's perspective at the start of this book, developed dental phobia in his twenties. That's when x-rays revealed a fully formed adult tooth in the wrong place. To move that tooth into its proper place, Ian needed surgery. He agreed to have his wisdom teeth removed at the same time.

Unfortunately, the surgery didn't go well, and Ian began avoiding the dentist altogether. That worked for about ten years, but by then Ian had a number of cavities that were starting to cause problems. It became a domino effect: he hated seeing the dentist, so he didn't go and his problems got worse. Finally, his wife convinced him to go, and he agreed—but only because he found a dentist who would give him nitrous oxide laughing gas.

That was many years before Ian became my patient, but he credits that experience as changing his life. Here's what he told me: "I remembered kids from my neighborhood talking about laughing gas and how they thought going to the dentist was fun. I thought maybe it could help me, so I found a dentist who used nitrous oxide. I told him about my past experiences and my fears. He said, 'Don't worry, you'll do great.'"

That dentist was right: Ian did do great. And now, as one of my patients, he continues to do so thanks to the many fear-free, pain-free options I offer.

Here's an overview of them:

## Distraction
*For those with minimal fear*

For many people, fear of the dentist can be eliminated by simply removing or masking the sounds and sights that cause distress.

Take the drill, for instance. Many people hate the very sound of it. While silent drills aren't yet available, many dentists offer high-quality headphones that filter out the sound. Tuning into your favorite radio station or the songs on your phone or MP3 player can further dampen the sound of the drill—and make your experience more enjoyable.

Certain music can also induce a state of relaxation. So can watching a favorite movie, which is why I offer DVD glasses. Shaped like a pair of ski goggles, these glasses, when combined with theater-quality sound, can make you feel as if you're watching a movie on a 50-inch widescreen TV. Dentists who offer these glasses typically have a large library of movies from which you can choose. You can also bring in your own DVDs.

## Nitrous Oxide Laughing Gas
*For those feeling more fearful or experiencing mild anxiety*

Nitrous oxide laughing gas may be a great choice if seeing the dentist causes you fear and mild anxiety. Clear and sweet-smelling, it aids relaxation and relieves minor pain. Although laws prohibit nitrous oxide laughing gas for initial exams (you must be fully aware for those), I routinely offer it to all my patients for everything else. What's more, I offer it for FREE. That's how much I believe in it!

Used as a dental anesthetic since 1844, nitrous oxide laughing gas is very safe. It, along with oxygen, is administered by your dentist through a small mask placed over your nose. Your dentist controls the amount of nitrous oxide laughing gas you receive, always keeping your comfort and safety top of mind. The goal is twofold: to help you relax, and to minimize your pain.

If you've never tried nitrous oxide laughing gas, you may be surprised at how far it can go in relieving your fear and anxiety. I tell people it takes the edge off, just like having a drink or two. While you will remain conscious throughout your appointment and remember it afterwards, the gas will make you so relaxed that you won't mind having your teeth cleaned. Many people also lose their fear of having local anesthetic, such as Novocain. As one of my patients says, "By the time you've administered the laughing gas, I hardly care what else you do."

Although the gas wears off quickly and there are no after-effects, most dentists will give you pure oxygen for five to ten minutes before sending you on your way. An added benefit of nitrous oxide laughing gas is that you can drive yourself to and from your appointment, which you cannot do with the sedation methods described on the next pages. You can also return to work, paint the garage, play the piano, or engage in other activities afterward, something you cannot do with other sedation methods.

## MAKE A WISE CHOICE

Nitrous oxide laughing gas typically costs $80-$100 per visit and is an out-of-pocket expense for most people, even those with dental insurance. But keep in mind that nitrous oxide laughing gas makes it possible to have more work completed during a single appointment, which can save you time and money over the long run.

Also keep in mind that while nitrous oxide laughing gas helps most people relax, it can very rarely have the opposite effect, making a small percentage of people feel anxious and perhaps even paranoid. So if you've never had nitrous oxide laughing gas before, be sure to tell your dentist. Also inform him or her about any bad reactions you've had in the past, whether to nitrous oxide laughing gas, Novocain, or any other anesthetic or medication.

You may also want to disclose other information. For instance, if a single pain pill knocks you out, *say so*. If you get loopy after drinking one glass of wine or nauseated after taking two aspirin, *let your dentist know*. Disclosing this information helps your dentist to decide how much medication to give you.

## Oral Sedation
*For those who feel mild anxiety*

If you've ever taken a sleeping pill, you've engaged in a form of oral sedation. Oral sedation dentistry is simply the use of oral medication to reduce your fear, anxiety, and pain so that you can undergo dental procedures. For most people who are sedated, time flies. What feels like just a few minutes could actually be six or more hours.

There's a range of oral sedation possible depending upon the dosage and each individual's response. At one end of the spectrum is a heightened state of relaxation during which you may fall asleep but be easily awakened. At the other end is a state of near unconsciousness after which you will remember little to nothing of your dental visit.

When orally sedating my patients, I generally prescribe a medication such as Valium. I instruct most patients to take one pill the night before their appointment, so they get a good night's sleep. Depending on how deeply sedated I want the patient to be (and taking into account his or her height and weight, as well as level of anxiety or fear), I may also advise taking a second pill approximately an hour before their appointment.

If you experience mild dental anxiety, oral sedation, which will affect you for two to three hours, may be a good option, especially if you're having a root canal. Oral sedation is both safe and effective, although it does come with a downside: once you've taken the pills, there's no way to increase the level of sedation, which means that if you aren't sufficiently sedated, you may end up feeling the exact anxiety you were hoping to avoid. If your anxiety is severe enough, your appointment may have to rescheduled.

### ARRANGE A RIDE

If you or your dentist opt for oral sedation, you must arrange for someone to drive you to and from your appointment. You cannot drive yourself.

## IV Sedation

*For those who experience acute stress or suffer from dental phobia*

With IV sedation, rather than taking a sedative at home, you receive it at your dentist's office, and rather than being delivered via a pill, it's delivered intravenously. One advantage of this is that it's fast acting; you'll be out in less than a minute. A second advantage is that your dentist can easily adjust the level of sedation. This means he or she can choose how sedated you are. You can, too. Some patients opt for feeling very, very relaxed, while others, particularly those who suffer from acute stress or dental phobia, prefer sleeping soundly through their entire appointment.

The big advantage of IV sedation is that you won't feel any pain (and in the rare instance you do, your dentist can quickly sedate you further).

If you need a lot of dental work, IV sedation often makes it possible to have it all done in a single visit. In fact, what I can do in six hours on a sedated patient would normally take me ten to twelve hours (five to six appointments) on someone who is awake.

### ASK QUESTIONS

When talking to your dentist about IV sedation, be sure to ask who will be administering the sedation medication, adjusting the sedation level, and monitoring your vital signs, including your pulse and blood pressure. Some dentists are certified to administer IV sedation themselves, while others choose to bring in a certified professional, most often a highly trained Certified Registered Nurse Anesthetist (CRNA).

If you have the choice, I always recommend choosing the latter option. That way, your dentist can concentrate on what he or she does best: providing high-quality dental care. In fact, even though I am board-certified to administer IV sedation, I choose to have a CRNA do so. That way I can stay completely focused on your dental care while the CRNA stays focused on everything else. This is the same model used in every hospital in the U.S.

Regardless of which sedation option you chose, ensure your safety by telling your dentist about all medications you take, including over-the-counter medications and herbal supplements, as well as all medical issues for which you are and have been treated.

Also let your dentist know if you've smoked marijuana or taken any other drugs. Your dentist won't judge or report you. Rather, he or she will use that information to keep you safe.

## IS SEDATION DENTISTRY RIGHT FOR YOU?

While many people think sedation dentistry is just for people with acute stress or dental phobia, others can benefit as well, including:

- **People who have a strong gag reflex.** Some people cannot tolerate even the smallest instrument in their mouths. If you're one of them, sedation dentistry can help you relax so you aren't bothered by the instruments or the treatment.

- **People who need extensive treatment.** Complex root canals, impacted wisdom teeth, and dental implants are just a few of the procedures for which you may wish to be sedated.

- **People who are busy.** If you feel pressed for time, you may want to opt for sedation, which can make it possible to complete your dental work in a single, extended appointment instead of multiple appointments spread over several weeks.

# CHAPTER 9

# Showing Up for a New Kind of Dentistry

*"Being brave isn't the absence of fear. Being brave is having that fear but finding a way through it."*

*— Bear Grylls, British adventurer, writer, and television presenter*

For many people fearful of seeing the dentist, one of the biggest challenges may be making—and keeping—appointments. You're likely to think, "Seeing the dentist has been painful in the past, and I don't want to repeat that."

Dentists and their staffs understand. Trust me. While you may be thinking that you're the only fearful person out there, you're not. Dentists actually care for people just like you every day. It's what we do. And some of us, me included, actually build our practices on caring for anxious, fearful, and phobic patients.

Here are some things a fear-free, pain-free dentist will do for you (or that you can ask him or her to do for you) before you even step across the office threshold:

- **When you call to schedule your appointment, share your fears and concerns.** Be as specific as possible. If walking in the door makes your heart race, say so. If the smell of the office bothers you, tell the person you're talking to. If seeing a needle makes you cringe, admit it. If you're worried that you may faint, acknowledge it. If you wonder what will happen if you need to go to the restroom, ask.

- **Ask for a ride.** My patient Ian often used to get within blocks of his previous dentist's office only to turn around and head back home. And he's not alone. Many of my patients say that one of the hardest things for them to do is get to their appointments. If getting to your dentist's office is a problem for you, ask a friend, family member, or work colleague to drive you. Also ask your dentist for his or her suggestions.

- **Ask for someone to escort you from your car to the office.** Some people have no problem driving to their appointments but just can't make themselves walk into their dentist's office. If you're one of them, when you get to the parking lot, call the office and say, "Hi. I'm here for my appointment, but I'm afraid to get out of my car. Can you help me?" You'll be pleasantly surprised at how fast someone will be out to get you and how helpful he or she will be.

## IDENTIFY YOUR TRIGGERS

"If you're afraid of the dentist, I encourage you to identify what triggers your fear. For instance, I know that the longer I sit in Dr. Shamblott's waiting room, the more panicky I feel. So I wait outside—in my car, on a bench, wherever. Then, when he is truly ready for me, I walk in, say hi, and climb into the chair. Within seconds, I'm getting nitrous oxide laughing gas to help me relax."
- *Ian*

- **Familiarize yourself with the office.** If you have time, ask for a tour of your dentist's office and what you can expect to happen during your appointment. Also check out your dentist's website, where you may find a virtual tour which allows you to get familiar with the dentist's office from the comfort of your own home.

## FIND OUT WHAT TO EXPECT

To see what you can expect during a typical appointment at my office, visit www.shamblottfamilydentistry.com/dental-fear.

- **Bring a security blanket.** Whether it's a literal blanket or a figurative one such as a stuffed animal (I have many adult patients who derive a great deal of comfort from their stuffed animals) bring what comforts you.

- **Know how you experience stress.** While I don't want to overgeneralize, men tend to sweat while women tend to get cold. Knowing how you experience stress can help you prepare for it. If you think you're likely to sweat, wear a T-shirt. On the other hand, if you're likely to get cold, bring a sweater or ask for a blanket.

- **Take your medication as prescribed.** Unless your dentist tells you otherwise, take your blood pressure and other medications as you normally would. If you typically get up and take medication before leaving the house, do so—even if your appointment is at 8 a.m.

- **Pay attention to what you drink.** If you normally get up and drink two cups of coffee to get yourself going, great. But if you've got a dental appointment and know you get anxious, you may want to skip the second cup in favor of eating a healthy breakfast. You don't want to be jittery or feel light-headed. That will just add to your upset. Limiting caffeine will also help prevent an increase in blood pressure or a sudden spike or drop in your blood sugar level (and prevent the need to stop your appointment for a bathroom break).

- **Eat as you normally would.** Unless you are undergoing sedation or are advised otherwise, eat meals (and snacks) as you normally would. Skipping them before an appointment can make you feel lightheaded, dizzy, or faint.

- **Pay ahead of time.** Ian hands my assistant his credit card before we even get started. That way, when his appointment is over, he doesn't have to wait around. He just grabs his card and his coat and walks right out the door.

- **Ask for stress balls.** Many people don't know what to do with their hands during an appointment. Some squeeze their hands so tightly they turn blue. Soft squeezable balls give hands something to do before and during your appointment.

# 10 | Mindset Matters

*"Nothing in life is to be feared, it is only to be understood. Now is the time to understand more, so that we may fear less."*
— *Marie Curie, physicist and chemist*

Like a lot of my patients, my friend Steve was forced to face his dental fear head on after developing a severe toothache. In Steve's case, it happened while he was on vacation in Panama. He spent many sleepless nights hoping the pain would go away. It didn't. In fact, it got so bad that he had to opt out of many of the vacation activities he and his family had planned.

Then, his sister-in-law, a dental assistant, came to visit. She told Steve his pain wasn't going to go away and that it would get worse the longer he delayed. She also told him that he was letting bad memories of dental visits ruin a perfectly good vacation.

Thanks to her tough-love approach (which may not work for everyone), Steve decided to make an appointment. But first, he had to find a dentist. "Panama is a country known for its health and dental care," says Steve. "But I didn't want to go to just any dentist. I wanted to find a dentist who would take my fear seriously. And one who would make sure I didn't experience any pain."

> *I didn't want to go to just any dentist. I wanted to find a dentist who would take my fear seriously.*

After talking to a number of Panamanians, as well as members of Panama City's ex-pat community, Steve went to see a dentist who came highly recommended. That's when he learned that he needed a root canal. In too much pain to put it off any longer, he agreed to have it done that very afternoon.

Steve found the root canal to be much easier than he had made it out to be in his mind. That's because he was fortunate to find a dentist with a fear-free, pain-free approach to dental care. "It was over in no time and was far less of an ordeal than I imagined," says Steve. What's more, the root canal gave Steve the confidence to get other needed dental work done. He even had his wisdom teeth removed, which enabled him to achieve his lifelong goal of getting braces. And although he readily admits that he still doesn't visit the dentist as often as he should, he's no longer afraid of doing so.

There's an important point to Steve's story I want to highlight: In his mind, he had made out the root canal to be much more difficult and painful than it actually ended up being. So many of our fears and anxieties arise from preconceived notions or scenarios we play out in our minds. This just emphasizes the importance of mindset in dealing with the realities in front of us rather than the myths in our heads.

## DENTAL REALITIES AND MYTHS

### REALITY OR MYTH?

Dental phobia is a real disease that affects millions of adults.

**Reality.** Nearly ninety-two million people in the U.S. are afraid to get the dental work they need.

### REALITY OR MYTH?

If I have a toothache, putting aspirin on my gums will relieve the pain.

**Myth.** Putting aspirin on your gums can damage them. Try clove oil instead. Available at most pharmacies, it's the most effective home remedy for tooth pain. But use sparingly as prolonged use can be nerve-deadening. And if your pain is severe or prolonged, wakes you up at night, or makes it hard to sleep, skip the clove oil and instead get to your dentist fast.

### REALITY OR MYTH?

Keeping my teeth and gums healthy with regular brushing may lower my risk of developing dementia later in life.

**Reality.** A University of California study that followed nearly 5,500 elderly people over eighteen years found that those who reported brushing their teeth less than once a day were 65 percent more likely to develop dementia than those who brushed daily.

### REALITY OR MYTH?

My parents had dentures at age fifty so I will, too.

**Myth.** With daily brushing and flossing and today's advanced dental care, your teeth can last a lifetime. Even people in their eighties and nineties now retain their teeth. But although the percentage of Americans needing dentures is declining by 10 percent a decade, they will still be needed by the more than thirty-seven million adults who are missing full sets of teeth today, according to the American College of Prosthodontists.

### REALITY OR MYTH?

Garlic relieves tooth pain.

**Myth.** Though garlic may keep you safe from vampires, it won't keep you from feeling the pain of a toothache. If you have a toothache, the best thing you can do is make an appointment with a fear-free, pain-free dentist right away.

### REALITY OR MYTH?

People can eat as well with dentures as they can with their real teeth.

**Myth.** Even the best dentures in the world operate only 15-20 percent as well as your natural teeth, making it difficult and uncomfortable to chew.

### REALITY OR MYTH?

If I have a cavity, I'll know it.

**Myth.** Mild decay doesn't cause symptoms, and most cavities aren't visible to the human eye. But even if you can't feel or see a cavity, have it filled. Allowing tooth decay to advance can lead to more costly procedures, such as root canals and crowns.

## The Quality of Your Beliefs

At the most fundamental level, the quality of your life, including the quality of your dental care, is determined by the quality of your beliefs. Your beliefs shape your thoughts, which in turn shape your actions, which ultimately shape the results you do—or don't—get. Which is exactly what Henry Ford once said: "Whether you think you can or can't, either way you are right."

I recently read a *Huffington Post* article that says the average person has about fifty thousand thoughts per day, and that 95 percent of those thoughts are repeated each and every day. I also read that at an amazing 70 percent of those thoughts are negative, meaning that we think more than thirty thousand negative thoughts a day.

And if even a portion of those thoughts is about bad dental experiences— real or imagined—no wonder anxiety starts to build. In fact, if we're not careful, our own minds can quickly become one of our worst enemies.

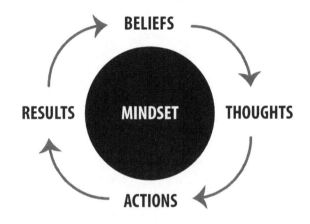

But that doesn't have to be the case. Instead, we can reprogram the beliefs that aren't serving us well. These beliefs are like weeds in a garden. They keep growing, and if we don't pull them, they will quickly overshadow all the beautiful flowers.

Staying positive can be a deed of daring for most of us, even on our best days. But for those who are afraid of the dentist or experience dental anxiety, staying positive can sometimes seem downright impossible. Having a positive attitude—about dental care and life in general—can go a long way toward ensuring we experience the good rather than just bad. That's because attitude plays a big role in determining how we feel about our experiences.

## Focus Pocus

Here's a little experiment. Choose one thing to think about right now but whatever you do, don't think about shoes. Don't think about the shoes on your feet, the shoes in your closet, or the shoes you saw while shopping last week. Certainly don't think about the shoes your kids are about to outgrow or the ones your favorite athletes wear. Think about whatever you want, just don't think about shoes.

Despite my instructions, what are you thinking about?

Shoes!

That's because trying not to think about something actually gets you thinking about it.

The next time you're at the dentist, rather than trying not to think about what's going on in your mouth, think about something else: how to drive home from your appointment, when to have your house painted, how to celebrate your parents' wedding anniversary. Directing your mind to the past or future by thinking about the goal you scored in high school or where you'll live when you retire can also help you distance yourself from what's going on.

Concentrating on a word, image, or object can also help distract your mind. If it's a word, choose a positive word such as warm, calm, safe, relaxed, or comfortable, then slowly spell out the word with your finger, sounding out the letters as you go. If it's an image, picture all the details as clearly as you can, everything from the angle of the sun to the length of the shadows, from the grains of sand to the different shades of green. And if it's an object, sense it resting loosely in your hand while you imagine the weight, texture, and shape of it.

This is also an ideal time to repeat an affirmation such as "I replace fear with confidence" or "I feel cool, calm, and completely relaxed." If distracting, negative thoughts arise, refocus your attention on your word, image, or object, breathing deeply all the while.

# 11

# Three Techniques for Achieving Calm

*"Calm mind brings inner strength and self-confidence, so that's very important for good health."*

— *The Dalai Lama, Buddhist monk*

Affirmations are one way to redirect your thoughts away from your anxiety and fear toward something more positive and affirming. To affirm means to "make firm" whatever you dream or imagine, including what you imagine happening during your dental appointments.

Writing down a few affirmations and saying them aloud to yourself before, during, and after your appointments can help you replace your negative thoughts with more positive ones. Repeating affirmations can also help you replace anxiety with confidence.

Here are some examples of affirmations that work well for my patients:

- "I like seeing my dentist."

- "I feel safe at the dentist."

- "Seeing my dentist and knowing I'm taking good care of my dental health makes me happy."

- "I feel a rush of confidence whenever I think about visiting my dentist."

- "I have healthy teeth and a beautiful smile."

- "I am in complete control of my life, even when I'm visiting my dentist."

Here are three ways to make your affirmations more powerful:

- **Stay in the present.** If you phrase your affirmations in the future, you'll always be waiting for the results. Instead, phrase them in the present. Say "I am enjoying a pain-free experience with my dentist," rather than "I will enjoy a pain-free experience with my dentist."

- **Stay positive.** Affirm what you want, not what you don't want. Say "I feel safe, comfortable, and relaxed when I'm at the dentist," not "I won't be afraid when I'm at the dentist."

- **Stay specific.** Affirmations are most effective when they're specific and meaningful to you. For instance, "I feel my mind and body relax the moment I kick off my shoes and settle into my dentist's blue chair" is better than "I feel relaxed at the dentist."

## THE POWER OF REPETITION

The more you repeat your affirmations, the more powerful they become. Be sure to say them as if you really mean them, thinking about each word and feeling its power. Say them aloud while waking up, getting dressed, driving the kids to practice, gardening, running, and falling asleep. You can also record affirmations on your phone and listen to them. It may sound corny, but it really works.

## Visualize Your Success

Visualization is another important tool you can use to manage dental anxiety and fear. There's nothing complicated about it, yet it enhances your concentration and harnesses the power of your imagination, making it possible for you to focus your attention on what you want rather than on what you want to avoid. What's more, you already know how to visualize. You do it every time you daydream.

Essentially, visualization taps the power of your imagination to help create your future. It's like having your very own movie and knowing that the entire plotline—including the amazing, awe-inspiring ending—is in your hands.

Not sure how to visualize? Here's how in two easy steps:

## STEP

### Get Comfortable
Pull the blinds, turn down the lights, and turn off the music. Sit or lie down in a quiet place where you won't be disturbed. Relax. Take three deep breaths, feeling your abdomen expand more each time. With each inhale, say "I am." With each exhale, say "relaxed." As you exhale, let your muscles go limp. Beginning with your toes and moving up to your scalp, feel your muscles relax one by one . . . a little more with each breath.

**I am . . . relaxed. I am . . . relaxed. I am . . . relaxed.**

Let all self-doubt and negative thoughts float away. With each exhale, feel them leave your body. See them getting smaller and smaller—so small that they eventually disappear.

## STEP

### Rev Up Your Imagination
Once you feel relaxed, take a deep breath and picture yourself walking into your dentist's office feeling just as cool, calm, and collected as you would feel taking a hot bath, having dinner with a good friend, or walking on the beach. Then, picture yourself being greeted by a smiling receptionist and calmly talking with her for a few minutes about the weather or the movie you saw last night. Perhaps see yourself laughing at a joke or sharing pictures of your kids or grandkids.

Then, imagine yourself calmly taking a seat in the waiting room. Perhaps you're glancing through a magazine or using your phone to chat with a friend or play a favorite game. When the hygienist calls your name, you smile, stand up, and walk over to him or her. Together, you walk to the examination room. As you do so, you take a few more deep breaths to help yourself relax even further.

When you reach the examination room, the hygienist helps you get settled by offering you some water, a pair of sunglasses to block out unwanted sights, or a blanket to keep you warm. You say thanks and ask if you can take off your shoes. You also ask for whatever else you need need: different music, more water, Vaseline for your lips, a signal you can use if you need your dentist to stop at any point for any reason.

Continue playing your mental movie. See yourself all the way through your appointment, then see yourself saying goodbye to your dentist and the front-office staff, walking to your car or the bus, entering your home, sitting down for dinner with your family, and telling them how well everything went.

Once you've watched your mental movie all the way through, play it a few more times. Keep adding details and then "make firm" your success by adding an affirmation such as, "I am so proud of myself for doing exactly what I set out to do," or "Gosh, seeing the dentist today was so much easier than I expected. I couldn't have asked for it to have gone any better."

Then, beginning with your scalp and moving down to your toes, breathe in your power, feeling yourself become more relaxed, more confident, and more determined to have a positive experience with each breath.

The more often—and the more detailed—you visualize your visit to the dentist, the more comfortable and confident you'll feel before, during, and after your appointment.

Visualize when you first wake up. Visualize while you're eating your meals, driving to work, and running errands. Visualize while you're falling asleep and when you wake up in the middle of the night. Visualize anytime you start to feel anxious or afraid. As with affirmations, the more specific you make your visualization, the more powerful it becomes.

## Relax

Another technique that can help you manage anxiety and fear is progressive muscle relaxation. It's a two-step process. First you tense the muscles in a specific part of your body, such as your neck and shoulders. Then you relax them. By tensing and relaxing your muscles in combination, you produce a greater feeling of relaxation than you would if you concentrated on relaxing alone.

Here's how to do it:

**1** Find a quiet spot, and get into a comfortable position. Close your eyes and relax as much as you can.

**2** Take a deep breath, hold it, and let it out slowly while thinking of a calming, positive word or thought. Repeat this word or thought a few times as you sink further into your chosen position.

**3** Beginning with one foot, curl and tense your toes as much as possible. Hold the tenseness for about five seconds. Then, relax your toes. Take a deep breath, and feel the tension disappear. Stay in this relaxed state for about fifteen seconds, and then switch to the toes of your other foot.

**4** Repeat this with each set of muscles, moving from your toes and feet to your calves, thighs, buttocks, stomach, shoulders, arms, hands, neck, face, forehead, lips, tongue, and jaw.

After you've tensed and relaxed all your muscles, relax your entire body. Breathe naturally, but deeply, all the while letting go of any tension. Enjoy the feeling of relaxation as it washes over you.

In the beginning, try to set aside fifteen minutes twice a day to practice. Then, once you get the hang of it, use this technique whenever you start to feel tense or anxious, whether you're at the dentist or not.

## RELAX, THERE'S AN APP FOR THAT

### BREATHE2RELAX

A portable stress management tool, this app teaches you how to breathe from your belly, a technique that has been taught for centuries as a way of helping people relax.

### BREATHING ZONE

Featuring a clinically proven therapeutic breathing exercise, this app comes with easy-to-follow voice instructions and calming sounds that help reduce your stress and anxiety within just minutes. The breathing exercise will also decrease your heart rate and lower your blood pressure.

### RELAX MELODIES

Whether you want to relax while awake or get a better night's sleep, this app can help. It features more than fifty sounds such as the ocean, birds, and rain. Set the timer, and it will stop playing. Set the alarm, and it will wake you.

# CHAPTER

## 12

# Dental Emergencies

*"Faced with the choice of enduring a bad toothache or going to the dentist, we generally tried to ride out the bad tooth."*

— *Joseph Barbera, animator*

Actor Johnny Depp once quipped: "Trips to the dentist? I like to postpone them." I guess that's why his teeth look the way they do.

If you're like Johnny and millions of other Americans, you also put off visiting the dentist. But if you do so for too long, you're likely to find yourself in need of emergency dental care. In fact, one in four Americans will experience a dental emergency at some point in their lives, many as the result of a sports-related accident.

Studies show that teeth-related problems play a significant factor in why kids miss school and adults miss work. According to the Centers for Disease Control and Prevention, 164 million work hours are lost each year due to dental issues.

*According to the Centers for Disease Control and Prevention, 164 million work hours are lost each year due to dental issues.*

Diana is one patient whose dental issues did cause her to miss work, but not nearly as much as she might have if she didn't have a dentist she trusted.

Like many of my patients, Diana isn't a big fan of dentists, and that's no secret to anyone who knows her. But just because she doesn't like dentists doesn't mean she doesn't need one now and again. In fact, "need" is what brought her to me most recently.

Diana was at a working lunch with a client when part of her tooth broke off. In the past, that would have triggered a great deal of alarm—and anxiety—for Diana. But she had been experiencing my fear-free approach to dental care for two years, so instead of panicking, she pulled out her phone and called my office. We got her in that very afternoon, and she was back at work the next morning.

"I knew you'd have me pain-free in no time," Diana told me. "Whether it's a routine or emergency visit, you always take care of me, and that's a big comfort for someone who doesn't like going to the dentist. And as much as I joke about how special you make me feel, I know you and your team take care of all your patients with the same love and attentiveness that I experience every time I walk in the door."

Jackie, another patient of mine, recently had her own dental emergency. Just two days before she was supposed to leave for a two-week vacation, she noticed some pain in one of her bottom teeth. While that could be a nightmare for anyone, it was especially so for Jackie, who admits to being anxious about a number of things, including seeing the dentist. So she did what a lot of my patients do: she hoped the pain would go away. When it didn't, she worked up the courage to call my office and make an appointment.

Even though it was my day off, I headed into the office so that I could see Jackie right away. As soon as I examined her, I knew she needed a crown and figured she would need a root canal as well. Jackie was dreading the entire ordeal, partly because of all the root canal horror stories she'd

> *Even though it was my day off, I headed into the office so that I could see Jackie right away.*

heard over the years. But as she told her neighbor afterwards, it turned out to not be as bad as she had expected.

One reason is because I gave her nitrous oxide laughing gas to help calm and relax her. That, combined with Novacain, kept her pain-free during her entire three-hour appointment. And perhaps most important, she remained pain-free her entire vacation.

And while Jackie's not eager to repeat the process, she has become an advocate for my fear-free approach to dental care. The day after she returned from her trip she brought in a friend who needed two teeth pulled and a root canal. Jackie told me she figured if I could relax her, I could do the same for her friend. I was happy to, but if Jackie and her friend hadn't known where to turn, they could have found themselves in pain for a lot longer.

Don't let that happen to you. Instead, start paying attention to what your teeth are saying: when a tooth hurts, it's your body's way of telling you that something is wrong and that you need to see a dentist. But if you don't have a dentist or are so afraid of going to the dentist that you can't make an appointment, your only option is to live with the pain.

Taking quick action is especially important as it can mean the difference between saving teeth and losing them. The first step is assessing the situation to determine whether you have a situation that can wait for normal business hours, a dental emergency that needs immediate attention in a dentist's office, or a medical emergency that requires an immediate trip to a hospital emergency room.

If you're unsure, a good first step is to call your dentist. Here are some questions he, she, or a staff person is likely to ask you:

- How long have you been in pain?

- Which tooth or area of your mouth is in pain?

- How painful is it?

- Is the pain sharp or dull?

- Does hot, cold, or pressure make it hurt?

- Does the pain keep you from sleeping?

- Have you taken anything for the pain? If so, what, how much, and when?

- Do you have any other symptoms? Fever, swelling, or chest pain, for instance?

If the pain is bad, here are some things you can do to help relieve it:

- Take an over-the-counter pain reliever such as Advil, Motrin, or Tylenol as allowed by your physician. (Do not take aspirin! It may increase bleeding. Also do not place any kind of pill against your gum; doing so may burn your gum and make things worse.)

- Rinse your mouth every hour or so with warm salt water.

- Apply an ice pack or cold compress to your cheek or the area that hurts. Apply it for twenty minutes, then let the area warm up for twenty minutes before once again applying the ice pack or cold compress.

- Avoid air travel. The change in air pressure may make your pain worse.

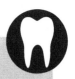

# WHEN TO SCHEDULE AN APPOINTMENT

If you experience any of the following, you should make a dental appointment:

- ✔ A loose tooth
- ✔ A tooth pushed out of position
- ✔ An injury to the tissue of the mouth
- ✔ Pain from wisdom teeth
- ✔ An abscess or infection

- ✔ A broken or cracked tooth
- ✔ A missing tooth
- ✔ Toothache
- ✔ A lost filling, cap, or crown
- ✔ A broken denture or partial

You should also make a dental appointment if:

- ✔ A tooth reacts to hot or cold food or drink and the pain lasts for more than a few seconds (if the pain lingers, it's a sign that you may have a cavity or need a root canal and a crown)

- ✔ A toothache or other tooth-related pain keeps you awake or wakes you up in the middle of the night

# CHAPTER 13

# Keeping Kids Fear-Free

*"Love is what we are born with. Fear is what we learn."*
— *Marianne Williamson, author and spiritual teacher*

Remember Andrew? He grew up with a mom who was terrified of going to the dentist. As a result, he himself grew up to fear—and avoid—the dentist. Renata also grew up with a parent who hated the dentist. No surprise that she hated going as well. But Renata was determined not to pass her fear on to her four kids who are now in their early teens and early twenties. Not one of them has any idea of the extent of their mother's dental fear, and that's something Renata takes great pride in.

If you're like Renata and are afraid of the dentist, you owe it to your children to keep your fear to yourself. While that may seem easier said than done, it's important that you don't let your own anxiety or previous dental experiences negatively influence those of your children.

If you worry that taking your child to the dentist could trigger your own anxiety and fear, take action ahead of time. For example, if sitting in the waiting room brings on a panic attack, ask the receptionist if you and your child can wait in the car until the dentist is ready. Or, if entering the office triggers your anxiety, call the receptionist from your car and ask him or her to meet your child in the hallway. Then return to your car, where the receptionist can call you when your child's appointment is finished.

Most fear-free, pain-free dentists and their staff will be more than happy to work with you to make sure the experience is positive for everyone.

But if, despite your and your dentist's best efforts, your child does seem fearful or apprehensive, here are some tips to help make dental visits easier:

## TIP 1

### Explain What to Expect

Just like adults, children fear the unknown. By explaining ahead of time what they can expect, you'll make dental visits easier—for them, and for you. For a step-by-step breakdown of what a child can expect in a typical appointment at Shamblott Family Dentistry, visit www.shamblottfamilydentistry.com/childrens-dentist.

## TIP 2

### Act Out a Pretend Visit

Before your child's first visit to the dentist, act out the experience. Allow your child to be both the patient and the dentist. Show your child how the dentist will count his or her teeth and use a mirror to compliment your child on his or her smile. Then, give your child a chance to brush his or her own teeth or the teeth of a favorite doll or stuffed animal. Then, reverse roles by giving your child the opportunity to examine your teeth.

## TIP 3

### Read Books about Visiting the Dentist

There are many books designed to get kids excited about seeing the dentist. Two of my favorites are *Curious George Visits the Dentist* and *How Many Teeth?* These and many other books are available in the waiting room of my office.

## TIP 4

### Downplay the Bad

Avoid words such as "cavity," "hurt," or "shot," which can make children feel afraid, even when there is nothing to fear. Instead, use phrases such as "The dentist is going to look in your mouth for sugar bugs," or "The dentist wants to count your teeth and check your smile."

TIP

### Time Your Visit
You know your children better than anyone, so be sure to schedule their dental visits for the time of day when your kids are at their best.

TIP

### Stay Calm
Even if your child works him or herself into a tizzy or starts acting out, stay calm. Do  not match your child's emotional state or lose your temper. Believe me, dentists have seen it all, and there's nothing for you to be ashamed of or embarrassed about.

TIP **7**

### Provide Support and Reassurance
Give your child positive feedback. Phrases such as "Great job" and "I'm proud of you for opening your mouth so wide" can go a long way toward building your child's confidence. So can physical feedback such as a hand squeeze or a shoulder or foot rub.

TIP **8**

### Offer Rewards
Talk to your child ahead of time about what you'll do after the appointment—a trip to the park or library, an extra hour of TV, or a favorite family meal. (One of the rewards for visiting my office is freshly made cookies, although I encourage you to think about rewards other than food.)

## LITTLE PITCHERS HAVE BIG EARS

Sooner or later, most kids ask, "Will it hurt?" They may have heard stories from their siblings or friends, or overheard adults talking about their own negative experiences. Even seemingly helpful statements such as "Don't worry, it won't hurt" can increase your child's anxiety, so choose your words with care. And never use the dentist as a threat or punishment by saying things such as, "You better brush your teeth, or the dentist will pull them out," or "If you don't floss, you're going to need fillings and they'll hurt." Statements such as these, even if they seem to go unnoticed at the time, can cause your kids to feel afraid the next time they visit the dentist.

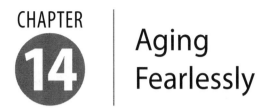

# CHAPTER 14

# Aging Fearlessly

*"Why is it that when we get older, we get more fearful?"*
— *Sandra Bullock, actor*

My patient Carol, now in her sixties, describes herself as having a "fairy tale life." She grew up in a close-knit family, traveled the world, and married a great guy with whom she lived happily for thirty-seven years. But despite her near-perfect life, Carol never got over her childhood fear of the dentist.

"As a kid, I had a lot of cavities," explained Carol the first time I met with her. "While I'm sure the dentists I saw back then did the best they could, they were always in a hurry. They never allowed much time for the Novocain to kick in. As a result, I was always uncomfortable or in pain."

The dentist Carol saw as a young adult was equally inattentive. He was also fond of pulling teeth. At one point a specialist he sent her to said, "I don't know why he wants your teeth pulled. You don't need them pulled." After that, Carol stopped going to the dentist altogether.

As the years passed, she became increasingly insecure about her teeth. "People used to comment on what a beautiful smile I had, but over time, they stopped commenting and I stopped smiling," said Carol. "I felt ugly. I also felt guilty. I knew I was supposed to get my teeth cleaned twice a year, and the longer I went without doing so, the guiltier I felt."

Carol kept promising herself that she'd make a dental appointment, but she didn't. Then she was diagnosed with Crohn's disease, an inflammation of the lining of the digestive tract which can lead to a sudden and urgent need to use the bathroom—even in the middle of a dental exam. Her diagnosis gave her one more reason to put off seeing a dentist, but it also made her realize the importance of taking care of her health, a message that hit home when her beloved husband died.

It took Carol nearly a year after his death to work up the courage, but she finally called my office to schedule an appointment. "I'm so glad I did," Carol told me. "You were very understanding of my fear and never made me feel bad about my smile, my teeth, or myself."

But what else helped? One thing that did was the nitrous oxide laughing gas I administered to help her relax. I also numbed her gums before giving her Novocain to ensure she wouldn't feel any pain.

A patient ever since, Carol experienced an a-ha moment during her most recent appointment. I came out of my office to find her talking and laughing with the billing coordinator. I said, "Well, that's something I enjoy hearing around here: laughter!" My comment made Carol realize that seeing me is no longer an experience she dreads, but one she looks forward to.

> **One in four Americans over age sixty-five has no teeth, according to the Centers for Disease Control and Prevention.**

One in four Americans over age sixty-five has no teeth, according to the Centers for Disease Control and Prevention. Many more have fewer than the adult standard thirty-two. These missing teeth can signify major health issues, such as diabetes and heart disease, both conditions that poor oral health can worsen. So if you're starting to lose your teeth, you owe it to yourself, your health, and your wallet to see a dentist. The sooner you do, the fewer problems you'll have, the less treatment you'll need, and the less expensive it will be.

As we age, we grow more mature but may still carry some—or even many—of the fears that frightened us as children: fear of heights, fear of snakes or spiders, fear of high places, and yes, fear of the dentist.

At the same time, many of us acquire new fears. Some of these are the result of physical changes. Take Susann, for example. Recently diagnosed with rheumatoid arthritis, she now has a hard time walking, let alone getting in and out of her dentist's chair. As a result, she sometimes feels trapped, which has increased her fear of seeing the dentist. And Anne, now nearly ninety, doesn't see or hear as well as she once did, which leaves her feeling anxious, especially when outside her comfort zone, which is exactly where she feels when she is at the dentist.

## EVEN DENTISTS CAN DEVELOP NEW FEARS

Even I'm not immune to new fears. Not long ago, in preparation for shoulder surgery, I had to have an MRI. I've had a number of them in the past, and none were a big deal. But this time was different. They slid me into the MRI tube, and I panicked. I felt like I was in a coffin and that I was suffocating.

I didn't last thirty seconds. I didn't even wait for them to slide me out. Instead, I climbed out. I was embarrassed, but then I did what I tell my patients to do—I asked for what I needed: an open-sided MRI machine. And while that wasn't a perfect solution, it did allow me to get the MRI completed comfortably.

Other changes also occur as we age. Our mouths get drier, for instance, mostly as a result of decreased saliva flow. This happens so gradually that many people aren't even aware of it. First, we may find ourselves getting up in the middle of the night to get a sip of water. Then, we may get up for a glass of water. Before long, we're taking a glass of water to bed with us— and getting up in the middle of the night to refill it.

This natural tendency toward a drier mouth is compounded for many older adults by the medications they take. According to Centers for Disease Control and Prevention statistics, more than 76 percent of Americans age sixty or older use two or more prescription medications monthly, and 37 percent use five or more. Many of these list "dry mouth" as a common side effect. And although referred to as "dry mouth," many people notice that their mouth isn't the only thing that's dry. Their lips, tongue, and throat may be as well.

Having a dry mouth can result in several dental-related problems. For instance, without the lubrication that saliva provides, you may have trouble chewing or swallowing your food. You may also worry about your favorite bread or spinach dip getting caught on or between your teeth. These problems can be made worse by the receding gums that also accompany aging.

But perhaps the biggest problem—at least as far as I and other dentists are concerned—is how reduced saliva flow affects your teeth. Because saliva washes your teeth and neutralizes the acid that causes decay, those who suffer from dry mouth are not only likely to get more cavities, they're likely to get them faster, which is why some people who have always had relatively healthy teeth can suddenly discover they have ten cavities. And if having one cavity makes you anxious, imagine the anxiety ten cavities can cause.

Another thing that happens is that our age catches up with us. Fillings and crowns don't last forever. As we age, they may need to be replaced, often with composites or crowns, which can fill us with fear at the same time they drain our bank accounts. Teeth don't last forever, either. So it's no surprise that the molars that served us well our entire adult lives suddenly give out with little to no warning, often requiring a substantial amount of work to repair or replace.

## DRINK WATER

If your mouth feels dry, taking frequent sips of water can help your teeth stay strong. So can oral moisturizers or saliva substitutes, which your dentist can recommend.

# 15

# Paying for Your Dental Care

*"The only thing that hurts more than having to pay for dental care is not having dental care to pay for."*
— *Bev Bachel, dental patient*

Financial stress can also cause pre- and post-treatment anxiety. If you're concerned about the financial cost of your dental care, talk with your dentist ahead of time as he or she may offer payment options and discount programs for patients without insurance.

If paying for your dental care is causing you anxiety, here are some suggestions:

**Understand Your Insurance**
If you have dental insurance, review your policy to make sure you understand the basics, including:

- **Your coverage.** Understanding your coverage means understanding what's covered, as well as any limitations or exclusions. For example, x-rays may be covered but be limited to one set every twenty-four months. Braces, on the other hand, may be excluded for anyone over the age of eighteen.

- **Your plan year.** This is typically a calendar year (January 1 through December 31), but not always.

- **Your preventive coverage.** Many plans cover one or even two cleanings and routine exams a year at 100 percent. Some only cover such cleanings and exams after you have met your deductible. Still others require coinsurance payments.

- **Your deductible.** This is the amount you need to pay out of pocket before your insurance will cover any of your dental care. Some plans do cover preventive care outside the deductible.

- **Your coinsurance.** Once you reach your deductible, your plan kicks in, paying a pre-determined percentage of the cost of your treatment. Generally, as when you see a doctor, preventive care is covered at 100 percent, while other treatment is covered at a lesser percentage: generally 80 percent for basic procedures such as fillings and root canals, and 50 percent for major services such as crowns or implants.

- **Your plan's annual maximum.** This is the maximum dollar amount your plan will pay toward the cost of your dental care each plan year. Any costs beyond this amount will be your responsibility. Most plans have an annual maximum of $1,000-$2,000 per person.

- **Your out-of-pocket costs.** These are the costs you pay for dental care. They include your deductible, any coinsurance payments, and any payments made after you reach your plan's annual maximum.

- **Your in-network vs. out-of-network options.** As when seeing a doctor, you can reduce your out-of-pocket costs by seeing a provider who is a member of your insurance plan's network. There's another advantage of seeing an in-network dentist: you typically don't have to pay the entire bill upfront. That's because your plan pays your dentist directly. You pay only your estimated portion. But even some out-of-network providers offer important advantages as well. For instance, I allow you to pay only your estimated portion and file the insurance paperwork for you, too.

## Find a Dentist Who's the Right Financial Fit

Finding the right dentist isn't just about finding a dentist with a good chairside manner. It's also about finding the right financial fit. Here are some tips for what to look for:

### Look for a Dentist Who Offers Financing Options

Many dentists offer financing options to help make dental care more affordable for those who don't have insurance. For example, I and thousands of other dentists offer programs such as CareCredit and Lending Club, which give patients a range of special financing options. In some of the programs, I even pay my patients' interest for the first twelve months, essentially giving them interest-free credit for an entire year. Other options—some that offer longer terms, some that are interest-bearing—are also available.

### Look for a Dentist Who Offers Free Services or Reduced Fees

As I already mentioned, when you come to my office, your first exam and first set of x-rays are free. You can also get free nitrous oxide laughing gas at every appointment (except the first, which is your initial examination).

### Look for a Dentist Who Offers Pro Bono Services

I am one of hundreds of dentists who participate in Dentistry From the Heart, a worldwide nonprofit organization that provides free dental care to those in need. Each year, I join fellow dentists and hygienists in helping thousands of men, women, and children get the dental care they need. We do so on the last Friday in February, while other offices do so on other days throughout the year. I also started Operation Open Wide, a program that provides free dental services on a Wednesday in July to veterans.

**Look for a Dentist Who Provides Estimates**

No one likes being surprised by how much something costs. People hate it even more when they think they're going to be charged one amount and end up being charged more. To protect yourself, ask your dentist to provide an estimate upfront. If you have dental insurance, you may want to submit that estimate to your plan and ask for a pre-determination of benefits. This enables you to know in advance which procedures are covered and the dollar value of that coverage.

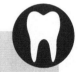

## ADMITTING YOUR FEAR PAYS OFF

"When I was in college, I needed my wisdom teeth removed. I couldn't afford to see the specialist my dentist recommended so I went to the University of Minnesota School of Dentistry. I was really scared, and I said so the minute I arrived, though I'm sure it showed. In any case, I was treated with a great deal of kindness and concern so even though I was paying considerably less than if I'd gone to a specialist, I felt I was still getting the best possible care."

*- Bev*

# Conclusion

*"A smile is a curve that sets everything straight."*
— *Phyllis Diller, comedian*

Susan never liked her teeth, which she considered too short and too gray. As long as she could remember, she wanted to have them crowned. She could even afford it, but she was too afraid. The idea of getting crowns just sounded complicated and painful.

But then Susan's mom, who had teeth exactly like Susan's, got ill. Shortly before her mom died, she told Susan, "Go get your teeth fixed. One of my biggest regrets is that I never did."

The very afternoon of her mom's funeral, Susan scheduled an appointment. Her goal: to have her teeth crowned within three weeks. But during her initial appointment, she learned what she had suspected all along— that getting crowns wasn't going to be quite so easy. She first needed a procedure that would require six months to heal.

That delay could have derailed Susan's plans, but she thought about her mom and made the decision to move forward. On the day her crowns were finally in place, Susan cried, not because she'd experienced any pain, but because she was so happy to finally have the smile she'd dreamed about her entire life. She faced—and beat—her fear.

Susan's story reminds me just how important dental health is—not only to our overall health, but also to our emotional well-being. There is a lot wrapped up in our relationship to our health and to our health care.

While getting past your fears may seem impossible, it's not. I see it happen every day to people like Susan, Amy, Andrew, Carol, Moira, Steve, and all the others you've read about in the pages of this book. And believe me, if they can do it, you can, too! All you need is a willingness to say "enough is enough" and a caring, empathetic dentist who practices fear-free dental care and offers you the following advances:

- Bonded, tooth-colored composite fillings that make teeth more resistant to fracture and breaking

- Antibacterial rinses that more effectively fight plaque and gingivitis

- Digital x-rays that use up to 90 percent less radiation and offer speed, accuracy, and the ability to see greater detail

- Digital impressions that are easier to administer than the goo-filled trays of the past

- Numbing spray that ensures pain-free Novocain injections

I'm excited about advances such as these and how more and more dentists are incorporating the kind of fear-free, pain-free dentistry I've talked about in this book. There is an alternative to being afraid. I'm happy to be a leader in the practice of it, and I urge you to schedule an appointment with me or with a fear-free, pain-free dentist in your area who can help you beat dental phobia—and live longer.

Still have questions? Visit www.shamblottfamilydentistry.com or call my office at 952-935-5599.

# Glossary

*"If you smile when no one else is around, you really mean it."*
— *Andy Rooney, writer and radio and television personality*

**Abscess.** A pocket of infection usually at the end of a tooth's root and often the result of a dead nerve in the tooth. The infection can quickly grow, spread, and become dangerous. If you think you may have an abscess, seek treatment immediately.

**Anesthesia.** The use of medication to prevent feelings of pain or other unwanted sensations. Dentists use Novocain and other similar medications to numb specific areas of the mouth so patients can comfortably undergo dental procedures. Some anesthesia medications are given in pill form; others are administered via IV. Anesthesia may also be used to deeply sedate patients so they are completely unaware of the procedure taking place.

**Bitewing x-rays.** Often referred to as "cavity-detecting," these x-rays show the upper and lower back teeth and how they touch one another, as well as the decay between teeth. They are taken inside the mouth.

**Composite fillings.** Tooth-colored fillings for small to medium-sized cavities. Used instead of amalgam or silver fillings to fill front and back teeth.

**Crown.** A lifelike, tooth-shaped cap that covers a tooth's entire above-the-gum surface. Tooth-colored (ceramic) or metallic (usually gold), crowns are used in place of missing or damaged teeth and to prevent teeth from cracking, fracturing, or breaking.

**Dental anxiety.** Feelings of fear or stress when thinking about or visiting the dentist.

**Dental bridge.** A false tooth or teeth with a crown on either side that is cemented together and used to replace missing teeth.

**Dental fear.** A fear of seeing the dentist, often caused by past experience.

**Dental implants.** A titanium cylinder or screw that is surgically placed in the jawbone to support a crown, bridge, or denture. Over time, the implant fuses with the jawbone making it an ideal long-term solution for missing teeth.

**Dental infection.** Also referred to as an abscess, a dental infection is a pocket of pus that has formed either at the tip of a root or in the gums. Serious infections may require a root canal and crown or even an extraction.

**Dental phobia.** An intense, unreasonable, and sometimes terrifying fear of seeing the dentist. Sometimes accompanied by panic attacks, this serious condition keeps millions of Americans from receiving dental care, often at the expense of their own health.

**Denture.** An artificial replacement of a full set of teeth, often supported by dental implants. Dentures are typically worn during the day and removed for sleep.

**Extraction.** Removal of a tooth from the jawbone. Extractions are performed for many reasons, including decay, infection, and impaction or because the tooth is cracked or it or its root is otherwise damaged.

**Fear-free dental care.** An emerging approach to dentistry that focuses on a patient's well-being and comfort.

**Gingivitis.** Red, irritated, and inflamed gums. With proper brushing, routine flossing, and regular visits to the dentist, gingivitis can be stopped before it becomes gum disease.

**Gum disease.** Advanced gingivitis. When gingivitis is left untreated, it infects the gum and eats away at the jawbone. If left untreated, teeth become loose and eventually fall out. Gum disease also increases risk of diabetes, heart disease, and stroke.

**IV sedation.** A sedative medication injected directly into a vein to help patients relax. IV sedation is one of the best ways to control the amount of sedation a patient receives. It's also one of the best ways to ensure patients feel no pain and have no memory of their dental procedures.

**Nitrous oxide laughing gas.** A harmless, sweet-smelling gas inhaled through a mask placed over the patient's nose. Patients feel relaxed but do not fall asleep or have amnesia. Offered free to all Shamblott Family Dentistry patients.

**Panoramic x-ray.** An x-ray that shows both the upper and lower jaws, and surrounding structures. Unlike bitewing x-rays, which are taken from inside the mouth, these x-rays are taken from outside the mouth.

**Partial.** A partial, removable denture used when only some teeth are missing.

**Sedation dentistry.** Sometimes referred to as "sleep dentistry," sedation dentistry uses oral or IV-administered medication to help patients relax, often to the point of being completely unaware of what is taking place.

**Root canal.** Used to remove diseased nerve tissue and replace it with a filling material called gutta-percha. Most teeth that undergo root canals will need a crown.

**Wisdom teeth.** Sometimes referred to as "third molars," the rear-most upper and lower teeth on both sides of the mouth. Wisdom teeth typically appear between the ages of seventeen and twenty-five, and often require extraction because there is insufficient jaw space for them to come in normally.

# Acknowledgements

*"No one who achieves success does so without acknowledging
the help of others. The wise and confident acknowledge this help
with gratitude."*
— *Alfred North Whitehead, English mathematician and philosopher*

I've wanted to write this book for a long time. I worked hard on it,
but I couldn't have done it without the help and support of many people.
I owe them all my gratitude and would like to thank the following people
in particular:

Kate Shamblott, for being the love of my life. Thank you for all you do to
support me and Shamblott Family Dentistry. Neither of us would survive
without you.

Rachel Shamblott, for being the best kid a dad could ever want. I am
so proud of you and all you've done to encourage other kids to visit the
dentist. Go Ray-Ray!

Dr. Claudia de Llano and Dr. Tracy St. Dennis, the associate dentists in my
office. Your commitment to fear-free, pain-free dental care is what sets our
practice apart.

Amy Knoll, my long-time dental assistant. The care and compassion with
which you treat our patients makes me proud, as does how willing you are
to help others overcome their fears by sharing your own.

All the members of the Shamblott Family Dentistry team. Thanks to you, coming to work is a joy. What's more, you brighten the lives of dozens of patients each day.

All those who agreed to be interviewed for this book. I appreciate your willingness to speak candidly about your own fear and anxiety in order to help others.

All my patients. The fact that you trust me with your dental care—and that of your families—means more than you can ever know.

# About Scott E. Shamblott, DDS, FAGD, FDOCS

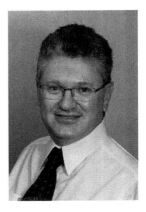

Dr. Scott Shamblott is a general dentist and the founder of Shamblott Family Dentistry in Hopkins, Minnesota. He focuses on fear-free dental care and has developed a worldwide reputation for his fear-free, pain-free approach to helping patients, particularly those with dental anxiety, fear, or phobia.

Born in New Ulm, Minnesota, he attended the University of Arizona, where he earned a Bachelor of Science degree in Finance. Dr. Shamblott then attended the University of Minnesota School of Dentistry, where he earned his Doctor of Dental Surgery (DDS) degree with high distinction. After dental school, he completed a general practice residency at the University of Tennessee Hospital in Knoxville, Tennessee.

In addition, he has earned a fellowship from the Academy of General Dentistry (FAGD) and from the Dental Organization for Conscious Sedation (FDOCS). He also attended the Medical College of Georgia to study IV sedation techniques and the Las Vegas Institute for Advanced Dental Studies to study sleep apnea.

Dr. Shamblott is a member of many professional organizations, including the Academy of General Dentistry, the American Academy of Dental Sleep Medicine, the American Academy for Oral and Systemic Health, the American Dental Society of Anesthesiology, and the Dental Organization for Conscious Sedation. A product evaluator for Clinicians Research, he is one of 450 dentists worldwide selected to test products and try out new dental tools, techniques, and materials.

He is certified in Advanced Cardiac Life Support and holds a Conscious Sedation Permit from the Minnesota State Board of Dentistry.

Dr. Shamblott makes frequent television and radio appearances and is an oft-quoted expert on issues pertaining to dental health. He has appeared on KSTP-TV Channel 5, Fox 9 - KMSP-TV, and KARE 11, and is a regular guest on Twin Cities Live. He was also the co-host of The Waiting Room on FM 107.1, a Twin Cities weekly radio program that covered all there is to know about dental health and other health care. Program podcasts are available on www.shamblottfamilydentistry.com.

Dr. Shamblott lives in the Twin Cities with his wife Kate and daughter Rachel. Kate helps with the office, and Rachel regularly appears with her dad on television, radio, and video, helping him connect with and communicate with children and teens about their dental health. Her message: take care of your teeth because they're the only ones you get.

# **Shamblott** Family **Dentistry**

Shamblott Family Dentistry is a fear-free, pain-free dental office located in Hopkins, Minnesota.

One thing that sets us apart from most other dentists is that we actually deliver on our mission statement, making sure we do everything we can to ensure patients have a positive experience. So whether seeing the dentist makes you smile or scares you to death, we offer:

- ✔ **FREE new-patient exams.** You shouldn't have to pay to find out what's wrong with your teeth, so your initial exam and x-rays are on us.

- ✔ **FREE new-patient emergency exams.** Just because it's an emergency, doesn't mean you should be charged outrageous fees, which is why initial exams and x-rays are free for new patients.

- ✔ **FREE nitrous oxide laughing gas.** You deserve to be comfortable and pain-free when visiting your dentist, so we offer free nitrous oxide laughing gas, even for routine cleanings.

- ✔ **FREE cookies.** To make your visits a bit sweeter, we offer fresh-baked cookies, as well as flavored coffees.

- ✔ **Same-day emergency visits.** If you have a dental emergency, we'll do our best to see you the same day you call.

✔ **IV sedation with a Certified Registered Nurse Anesthetist.**
For the ultimate in fear-free dental care, we offer IV sedation,
which induces such deep relaxation that most patients have little
to no memory of their visit.

✔ **Extended hours.** We're open early mornings, evenings, over the
lunch hour, and on Saturdays.

Part of what also makes us special is our unique fear-free, pain-free
approach to dental care:

✔ We focus on your wants and needs and will do all we can to make
you comfortable and pain-free.

✔ We use the most advanced tools, techniques, and materials.

To schedule an appointment with Dr. Scott Shamblott or one of the other
Shamblott Family dentists or to learn more about Shamblott Family
Dentistry, call 952-935-5599 or visit www.shamblottfamilydentistry.com.

## LIVE OUTSIDE MINNESOTA?

If you live outside Minnesota and are having trouble finding a fear-free,
pain-free dentist, give us a call. We see many patients from across the U.S.
and as far away as Europe and the Middle East and will work with you to
accommodate your travel schedule.

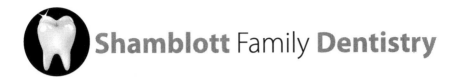

**Shamblott** Family **Dentistry**

Dr. Scott Shamblott has been seen and heard on:

- ✔ Twin Cities Live
- ✔ KSTP-TV Channel 5
- ✔ Fox 9 - KMSP-TV
- ✔ KARE 11
- ✔ Channel 12 Northwest Community Television
- ✔ myTalk 107.1
- ✔ KOOL 108 - KQQL 107.9
- ✔ Cities 97
- ✔ The Waiting Room
- ✔ Star Tribune Newspaper
- ✔ Sun Sailor Newspaper